T0197135

Defeat *Diabetes* Now

Defeat *Diabetes* Now

ALAN NEMTZOV RN

authorHOUSE®

AuthorHouse™
1663 Liberty Drive
Bloomington, IN 47403
www.authorhouse.com
Phone: 1 (800) 839-8640

Published by AuthorHouse 09/14/2015

ISBN: 978-1-5049-2705-5 (sc)
ISBN: 978-1-5049-2704-8 (e)

Library of Congress Control Number: 2015912486

Print information available on the last page.

This book is printed on acid-free paper.

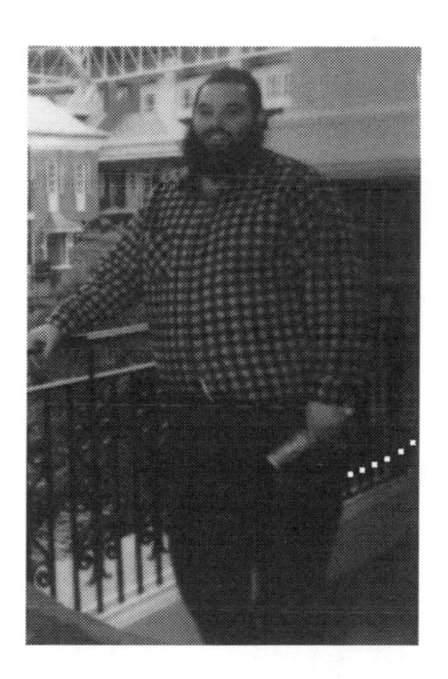

This was me in 2004; weighing 312 pounds, and taking 9 anti diabetic pills a day. I was living a miserable, difficult, unhealthy and unhappy life.

Acknowledgement

The Nursing Staff at Rockland Community College, especially Mrs. Eichers RN, MSN and Mrs. Schachter RN, MSN for their outstanding support, always going the extra mile.

Zev Goldstein, Esq. for his final editing and continuous support.

My parents, for raising me, and always believing in me, even when I didn't believe in myself.

My children, for their love and patience.

My wife Bernice, for being my inspiration, my guiding light and my partner for life.

Lastly my God, for constantly accepting and loving me as I am.

Table of Contents

INTRODUCTION

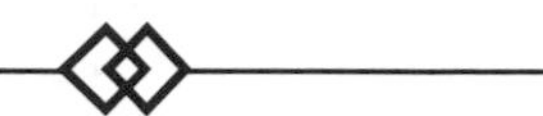

Diabetes is not a new disease; it was one of the first diseases described in ancient world cultures. Both Type I and Type II are chronic conditions that usually cannot be cured. All forms of dia-betes have been treatable since insulin became available in 1921, and Type II diabetes may be controlled with medications

Diabetes is affecting increasing numbers of people in Western civilization. Dr. Jeffrey Koplan of the Centers for Disease Control and Prevention (CDC), reported in October 2000 that diabetes was reaching epidemic levels in the United States. By 2011 the CDC estimated that nearly 26 million Americans have this incurable, but treatable, disease.

Modern medicine has not yet been able to develop a cure, or even to get a handle on ameliorating the devastation caused by diabetes. I believe that something is missing in the treatment of diabetics.

The present work posits the question: what is happening in our society that has lead to the explosive growth of the diabetic population, and how can we slow this trend down?

It is the purpose of this book to propose an answer that has worked for me, an answer that has worked for countless others with whom I've been able to share my experience.

How was I, a type II diabetic, able to shed my five medications (nine pills a day) for over eight years while maintaining normal blood glucose levels? What is lacking in diabetic treatment, what is the neces- sary link that connects all the dots?

I discerned the missing component while in nursing school: lifestyle changes which reduce the level of cortisol, also called the stress hormone.

This book will educate diabetics, explaining the sources of the disease, illustrating the consequences of diabetes, and promoting the lifestyle changes necessary to maintain normal blood glucose levels. Hopefully, you too can live life totally medication free.

It is my hope that practitioners too will utilize this innovative therapy when treating their patients.

No one has yet found a cure for diabetes, but I do believe that with your help we can prevent many of the unnecessary complications and deaths caused by diabetes.

God Bless, Alan Nemtzov, RN

CHAPTER ONE

AWARENESS

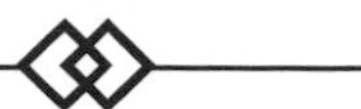

What a concept! Five years ago, if someone had told me what I'm about to tell you, I would have ignored the idea. Or I would have said, "Yeah, sounds great, but not for me." That was how I reacted to any positive or successful idea. It may be great for you, but count me out. It ain't going to happen for me. I was a statistic – the unlucky forty-year-old five-foot ten-inch tall shlub who weighed three hundred and ten pounds, with a blood sugar of two hundred after taking my five medications daily, totaling nine pills.

I had been on every diet imaginable since I was thirteen. The youngest of four, I was constantly ridiculed by my parents, older siblings, and friends. "What's the matter with you? Can't you just control yourself?" I ate like a lunatic just to feel some joy in my life.

When I got my driver's license @ age 16, my car was my sanctuary. I would polish off an entire pizza in the car by myself. *What an accomplishment*, I thought. Isolating myself in the car - finishing bags of chips, peanuts, Resse's, and other garbage on the way to any destination – was a great joy. Food was my friend, or so I thought.

Then the crap hit the fan. At age thirty-three, life wasn't going so well. A job usually didn't last more than a year, so benefits were typically out of the question.

I was living on food stamps and Medicaid, trying to raise a family of eight, and I had run out of job ideas. So I applied to become a taxi driver.

The livery-driving license required a blood test. I was peeing a lot at night and during the day, and I was constantly thirsty. I feared diabetes was the culprit, since both my aunt and grandfather had died from the disease.

My fears were confirmed, the glucose test came back positive: three hundred and thirty two. The doctor told me I'd have to test my blood sugars daily, take medication at certain times, go to a nutritionist, visit an eye doctor annually, and lose weight. I hated being told what I must do or couldn't do, or what I should eat or not eat, but the fear of dying young shook me up. I figured I'd just take pills for a few months and that would take care of it. Maybe I was making too big a deal of the whole thing.

Soon, I got really annoyed. I was taking the medications, but my symptoms were not subsiding. So, I had a great idea: stop the meds. Ingenious. I'll show that doctor who's in charge! I'll lose weight and everything will be just ducky. So I did. I dropped down to two hundred and sixty. *Perfect.* I was cured. Those doctors, what do they know anyway? No more meds, I told myself. But the inevitable happened, and I gained my weight back.

I was so miserable that I decided to go back to the doctor. He was gracious and increased my medications, told me to lose weight, to come back and see him in three months, and that was it. However, I wasn't doing well emotionally. Before each visit to the doctor, the fear of being scolded would set in. I would eat healthy for two days, or maybe one day, or perhaps, just *that* day. Then, when he didn't yell at me, off to Dunkin' Donuts I'd go.

This was not a life, but for me it was the only life I knew. I never imagined that there was a solution to all this insanity – that a life much different and more wonderful than the one I had been living was not only possible, but, could be my reality - that the answer to all my problems actually lay within me.

My experience to that point in my life had shown me the opposite: that I had no answer within me. Playing the victim child, blaming everything and everybody for my lack of success: that was the only life I had ever known how to live.

I was miserable. Self-pity and fear were my constant companions. They were the driving forces of my life. Happiness could only be found through food, the same food that was actually killing me - an obese diabetic - with every bite. The damage I was causing myself was far greater than I imagined. Not only was I dying physically, but I was also an emotional wreck.

The first light bulb went on in my head during the most unusual circumstance. I do believe God has a sense of humor. Once, while I was driving my taxi, a passenger complained to me about waiting twenty-five minutes for the car (me) to arrive. I told her that although I felt bad for her, her little calamity was nothing compared to my life. Once again, I was complaining to somebody else about my past. She didn't seem too interested, but it did shut her up.

I took a look at her in the rearview mirror and then twisted it so I could look at myself. I was disgusted at what I saw and what I had become. I said to myself "*you idiot. Look at yourself –driving a taxi fourteen hours a day, blaming everybody else about any problem you have ever had, going from one job to the next - a worthless nothing, that's what you are. You are to blame, nobody else. You are the one with the big mouth, always having to be right no matter what the consequences.*"

I have since learned that I can choose to be right, say "my" piece and risk be challenged with an argument. This attitude towards life leads to stress, which, for a diabetic like me, is akin to eating pure sugar.

On the other hand, I've learned a better, live-giving choice: to be happy with whatever life is giving me at the moment. I never was able to change the world with my big mouth; complaining always led to me being left unsatisfied. Either I got my way or I lost the argument, but in either case, the let down afterwards was always the pits.

This awakening in my taxi, that I didn't have to always be right, as painful as it was at the time, turned out to be the beginning of my new found life. It was the beginning of a search that is still in progress and gets more exciting as time goes on. The things I have learned about myself, my capabilities, and life in general, are extraordinary. Today I am *Awesome Al*, instead of Miserable Alan. When somebody asks me today, "Hey how ya doin?" I respond, "Awesome," and I mean it. It has proved to be a great source of joy to others, as well as being a consistent bulkhead against negativity in my own life.

The intention of this book is exactly this: to show you, no matter where you are in your life, a way to reach lofty levels of living that you never imagined possible.

No matter where you are with your diabetes, or with your weight, no matter what your age, creed, color, religion, or gender, you deserve and can have a better life.

I'm talking about an improvement in every aspect of your life: most importantly with your health, but also with your finances, with your relationships, and with your self-esteem. If money is your problem, the solution already exists. This book will also help you improve your current relationship, or perhaps to help you to find a significant other. The answer to all your dilemmas and calamities already exists. The challenge is to find that solution, and that is exactly what I plan to show you.

This is not a quick fix, it's not a "pop a pill and get cured" solution. Those things never seem to work. Time and again I have proven this to myself. The transformation from a miserable life to an awesome life takes time, perseverance, and patience. But that wonderful life will come, *guaranteed,* if you follow the suggestions in this book.

One of the difficulties I've had in my own recovery (and which I have seen in others' recovery as well) is that a quick fix approach *does* give moments of satisfaction. The quick fix *does* provide a modicum of instant gratification. However, the long-term approach I have experienced and offer to you here has far better and far longer-lasting results, even though it rarely provides that instantaneous high.

For me, I was often crushed by the frustration of waiting for recovery to catch. Taking the "right actions", without any of the promised results was so demoralizing.

The instantaneous high of the ineffective quick fix approach blinded me to the reality that the real solution has to be given a chance to work. I didn't get ill in a day; it will take more than a day to get well. Think exercise: its takes so long (weeks of dreary repetition) before you see the benefits start to kick in. The silver lining is that the solution offered here does work. It did for me, and it will for you. The power to defeat, well at least control, diabetes is within you, me, and each one of us.

I would love to credit myself by saying that courage and willpower were the driving forces behind my growth and recovery. But this would be an outright lie.

The truth is that pain, which seemed to be my nemesis, actually proved to be my friend. It was that pain of frustration that drove me to self-awareness and the willingness to change. My ability to even hear that still voice within, so deep and so quiet, was produced through pain. A lot of pain: the pain of hopelessness, the pain of loneliness, and the pain of despair. That awful feeling that, while life may be great for others, it won't be great for me. The pain that this is the way life is meant to be for me, and that this is how my life will always be, and never better, and that's it. That pain finally gave me suicidal thoughts.

I didn't need much convincing that my way wasn't working. I lived the "if only" life. *If only* my wife would stop nagging me, *if only* I was skinny, *if only* I had different parents, *if only* I had a better job, *if only* I were rich, and so on, then I would be happy. I just wanted my fifteen minutes of fame and never got it. My misconception about myself was so deep (I blamed everybody else for all my mishaps in life), that I was always under the impression that something other than me had to change in order for me to be happy.

The turning point for me was when I realized that the solution to all my problems was not from any external source. I was the source of my happiness. When I finally understood this concept, I was so relieved.

I thought I needed to change the world and my circumstances in order to be happy. The only thing I needed then, and still the only thing I need today to be happy, is to change myself. Even more than that, I finally understood that I actually have that power implanted in me, just as it is implanted in each and every human being to make that change a reality.

Wow! This was great news! A huge load had been lifted from my shoulders. That huge mountain I had created for myself and my problems now became a molehill. I don't need to change any *thing* in my life today or ever, to achieve happiness. I can be happy with myself *by* myself, and I actually have the power to achieve this.

It doesn't matter what my personal experience or situation is, or what my talents are. I can do this and live happily for the rest of my life. Sound like a fairytale? Really, it is paradise, and I actually live this way, as do many of my friends who live with the same ideals. The best news is: you can, too.

This is the truth that I want to give to you. This truth, this vision for a life in paradise, is the seed of hope that I pray to give to you in this book. This truth, that I have the power to be happy with myself *by* myself, is as much a reality for me today as is the truth that the sun rises daily in the east and sets daily in the west. I live this life today, and have lived it for the last four years. Strangely enough, it keeps getting better every day.

I never fantasized in my wildest dreams such a reality. It's like living in heaven here on earth. My life has changed radically for the better. It has gone from no hope, to going to school and becoming a nurse. I am truly humbled by the grace I have been blessed with. I feel compelled to pass on to others that which was given to me.

At this point you may be asking yourself, "*What do I have to do, and what does all this stuff have to do with my diabetes*?"

Well, learning how to live with diabetes is a process, and if you're reading this, you are well on your way to success. You have already begun to grow. The seeds have already been planted for your ultimate happy and healthy life. If you're anything like me, you're at a stage in your life where the old way is just not working. I couldn't take it any longer, and I was ready to hear another opinion about my life. As I said earlier, I didn't like being told what to do. I was Mr. Right. But this Mr. Right had to admit that I was very wrong. Are you ready to grow?

CHAPTER TWO

The Disease

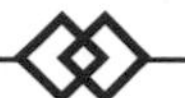

I found out that there was something wrong in the way I was thinking, or in the way I reacted to life, or both. I realized that my judgmental thinking caused me to overreact to life. My stinkin' thinkin' wasn't just affecting my sanity, but it was also hurting my health. You see, I am afflicted with the disease of diabetes, and judgmental thinking generates stress, which exasperates the etymology of diabetes.

I thought if I could only figure why or how my judgmental thinking was destroying my body and my life, I would have the answer to all my problems. The million–dollar question: Why was I overreacting, and how can I learn to cope in healthy ways? We will focus on this subject in detail later, but it's important to first focus on the issue that brought you to this book: diabetes.

What is this horrible disease that has become an epidemic and is killing so many people today?

Diabetes is a disease that is defined by elevated blood glucose levels. Diabetics are unable to maintain normal blood glucose levels.

Glucose is the major source of energy for the body. In order for glucose to provide this energy to the body, it needs to get into the cells. A hormone called insulin, which is produced and stored in the pancreas, is the necessary vehicle needed to transport this glucose through the bloodstream. Think of insulin as the Mail Man and the glucose as the mail; insulin is responsible for delivering the glucose from the bloodstream to muscle, fat, liver and most other cells so that our body can use it for fuel.

In a well-functioning body, the insulin is triggered through a thermostat-like system. When glucose is in the body, a message is sent to the brain to tell the pancreas to release insulin so that the glucose can either be absorbed by the cells for energy or, if there is excess glucose, to store it in the liver to be used when needed. As long as there is glucose in the bloodstream, insulin will make its deliveries. When all the glucose in the body has been absorbed, the brain tells the insulin to go back to the pancreas and not to come out again unless more glucose needs to be transported around. This cycle is repeated many times during the course of a person's day. Every time a person eats something, especially carbohydrates, this process occurs.

This is what happens when a person has a well-functioning body. However, a person with diabetes has difficulty in reducing the glucose due to various factors, paramount is the lack of, or dysfunction of, insulin.

The Type I diabetic, or "insulin dependant" diabetic, does not have sufficient insulin in the pancreas. The body destroys its own beta cells in the pancreas that produce the necessary insulin. Typically (there are exceptions) a person is born with this disease.

For the Type II diabetic, the production of insulin is not usually the problem. The pancreas often produces plenty of insulin. In fact, most Type II diabetics produce more insulin than non-diabetics.

The reason for this is that the pancreas tries to compensate for the elevated blood sugar levels, and therefore increases the production of insulin, a condition called *hyperinsulemia*. If left untreated and reaches extreme levels it could be as fatal as a hypoglycemic (low blood glucose) crisis.

A Type II diabetic is an "insulin resistant" diabetic. Insulin resistant means that the body's cells receptor sites don't adequately accept the insulin's delivery of glucose. This leaves the cells hungry, as well as leaving non-metabolized glucose in the blood (hyperglycemia).

Here are some other important contributing factors that exist in Type II diabetics.

1) There might be an unwarranted increase in glucose production in the liver, due to unbalanced insulin levels. This would confuse liver secretion of glucose, part of the thermostat system.
2) A decrease in the transport of glucose to the cells by insulin, either because the receptor sites themselves do not properly receive the glucose from the insulin (the mail box is missing or defective) or because of post-receptor defects within the cells themselves: the glucose which is delivered to the mailbox doesn't get utilized by the cells.
3) Impaired beta–cell function, which can also impair the release of insulin in response to high blood sugar levels; the beta cells in the pancreas are the insulin production site in our body.

Ninety–five percent of the people diagnosed with diabetes are Type II. We are, therefore, going to focus on the Type II diabetic, even though a lot of the remedies pertain to any diabetic, no matter the type.

Today, many Type I diabetics are developing Type II complications as well. They give themselves insulin shots for their lack of natural insulin. Yet, the insulin delivery system is being resisted by the cells, just like the Type II; usually due to obesity.

The Type I diabetic is usually born as such and can never recover and live without treatment, such as daily insulin shots, via a needle or insulin pump unless a successful pancreatic transplant takes place.

On the other hand, a Type II diabetic, which may also be a hereditary condition, though more difficult to treat, can eventually recover and live without any outside treatment, such as I do. It is possible to prevent an increase in blood sugars through a specific lifestyle that we will talk about later.

First let's take a closer look at what happens with the diabetic, when he or she consumes food. The food enters the body, is metabolized, and the brain messages the pancreas that insulin is needed in order to transport glucose into the cells. The pancreas secretes the insulin; however, the receiving cells are not able to accept the insulin. The cells therefore don't absorb the needed glucose and the cells are left hungry.

With time, they become really hungry for glucose. The glucose is in the body, but they just can't get it.

To visualize this, let's think: car. If the fuel pump is blocked, or is malfunctioning, then even with a full tank of gas, the car cannot drive. The insulin is like the fuel pump, and the glucose is the fuel. For the diabetic, when the insulin malfunctions, regardless of the reason, the cells cannot get their fuel, the glucose.

So they scream to the brain, "We need energy. Help!" The brain, in the interest of self-preservation, (which is its primary purpose), sends a message to both the liver and the stomach. It tells the liver to release some of its stored glucose into the body. The liver complies and releases the glucose.

More insulin is also released to make its glucose deliveries, but since the diabetic's system isn't functioning properly to transport the glucose into the cells they don't get fed.

The cells call the brain, "Hey! What's going on, where's my glucose?" The brain consults with the liver, and the liver tells the brain, "I'm doing all I can, if this keeps up, I'll run out of stored glucose". "Now what" asks the brain? "I know, I'll tell the stomach to have some hunger pains, signaling to the person that he needs to eat." The person then complies and eats. Once again there is more glucose in the blood, which also can't enter the cells.

The solution is to eat more, so he eats more and more and more. This is why one of the symptoms of diabetes is unsatiated hunger. The more he eats, the more the blood sugar levels increase. The brain keeps telling him to eat more since there still is a lack of glucose in the cells.

The more he eats, the hungrier he gets. The hungrier he gets, the more he eats. The more he eats, the fatter he gets. The fatter he gets, the less the insulin works due to adipose tissue (fat tissue) in the abdomen. While all this is happening, the diabetic just keeps eating, elevating the blood sugars higher and higher. Get the picture? Ouch.

This horrible cycle continues for years on end, without the diabetic even realizing that there is a problem. Pretty scary stuff if you ask me.

Furthermore, the consequences of being hyperglycemic (excess blood sugar) for any lengthy period of time are the same in both types of diabetes. *The body doesn't care why it is in a state of hyperglycemia.* The damage, regardless of the cause, is irreversible.

Both Type I diabetes and Type II diabetes create multiple health risks, such as blindness, loss of limbs, and kidney failure. Furthermore, damaged blood vessels result in poor wound healing which cause the loss of lower limbs. It also can cause heart malfunction, which among other things reduces blood circulation. Over time, this can also lead to heart attack, stroke, coma, and death.

There are two major types of complications associated with diabetes. The first type is "macro-vascular" (large blood vessels). This results from changes in the medium to large blood vessels. The blood vessels thicken and become occluded due to the plaque that adheres to the vessel walls. Eventually blood flow is blocked and can result in heart attack, stroke, or other peripheral vascular disease (which refers to pathology to any of the blood vessels outside of the heart or brain, such as the arms, legs, or other internal organs).

The second type of complication is "micro-vascular", affecting the small blood vessels. Retinopathy, nephropathy, and neuropathy, are the three major complications connected with micro-vascular disease. Retinopathy affects the retina in the eyes. Nephropathy affects the kidneys. Neuropathy affects small blood vessels that supply nerves.

The first complication we will discuss briefly is diabetic retinopathy. Hyperglycemia (increased blood glucose levels) causes thickening of the basement membrane, leading to incompetence, or weakness of the structure, of the vascular wall.

These damages change the formation of the blood-retinal barrier and also make the retinal blood vessels become more permeable. In simple language, they create tiny holes in the blood vessels. Small blood vessels, such as those in the back of the eye, are especially vulnerable to increased levels of sugar. As new vessels are formed they bleed and may even hemorrhage causing blurred vision.

At first, this may go unnoticed leaving just a few blood spots floating around the eye, causing minor changes in vision that will disappear after a few hours. It may seem that there is a small piece of dust in the eye. However, with time it gets worse and can cause blurred vision and eventually blindness. The longer a person has diabetes, the higher the risk of developing some ocular problem. Between forty and forty-five percent of Americans diagnosed with diabetes have some stage of diabetic retinopathy.

The next complication is nephropathy. The earliest detectable change in the course of diabetic nephropathy is a thickening in the glomerulus, which is in the kidney. This tiny ball-shaped structure, composed of blood vessels, is actively involved in the filtration of the blood to form urine. At this early stage the kidney may start allowing more albumin (plasma protein) than normal in the urine, something called albuminuria. Testing the urine for excess albumin is a common diagnostic tool used to detect diabetes.

As one's diabetes progresses some of the symptoms of nephropathy that may be found are: high blood pressure, unexplained weight gain, and swelling - typically the eyes are affected in the morning, and later in the day the lower extremities: legs, ankles, and feet.

Complications of chronic kidney failure are more likely to occur earlier, and progress more rapidly, when it is caused by diabetes rather than other causes. Even after initiation of dialysis or after transplantation, people with diabetes tend to do worse than kidney patients not afflicted with diabetes.

The last and most severe complication of diabetes is neuropathy. Blood vessels depend on normal nerve function, and nerves depend on adequate blood flow. With the decrease of blood flow due to vasoconstriction (constricted veins caused by macro-vascular disease), the nerves are not able to function to capacity.

Diabetic neuropathy affects all the peripheral nerves: pain fibers, motor neurons, and autonomic nerves. Therefore, it can affect all organs and body systems. There are several distinct syndromes based on the organ and the system affected, but these are by no means exclusive. A person can have sensorimotor and autonomic neuropathy or any other combination.

Some of the symptoms that may develop include: numbness and tingling of extremities (fingers and toes), erectile dysfunction, decreased or lost sensation to a body part, urinary incontinence, dizziness, impotence, to name just a few.

Decreased blood not only affects the nerves, decreased blood flow also affects wound healing, and normal functioning of bodily tissue. Cells will die without adequate blood flow, since our blood is the major transporter of nutrients and oxygen to the cells throughout the body.

Furthermore, a diabetic may have greater potential risks and/or complications due to their diabetes, should they acquire other disease.

The difficulty in treating diabetes is that it is a disease of slow progression, and can be quite asymptomatic (without symptoms) for many years.

According to the American Diabetes Association, there are an estimated 23.6 million children and adults in the United States who have diabetes, or 7.8 percent of the population, While an estimated 17.9 million have been diagnosed, 5.7 million people are not even aware that they have the disease. Moreover, 57 million people are pre-diabetic.

If present trends continue, one in three Americans (and 1 in 2 of minority populations) born in 2000 will develop diabetes in their lifetime. Each day, approximately 4,384 people are diagnosed with diabetes.

In 2007, 1.6 million new cases of diabetes were diagnosed in people age twenty years or older.

Diabetes is the fifth-deadliest disease in the United States. Since 1987, the death rate due to diabetes has increased by 45 percent. By contrast, death rates due to heart disease, stroke, and cancer have declined in the same period.

The primary focus for us diabetics is to maintain normal blood sugar levels as much as possible in order to prevent any of the complications caused by diabetes. The reason for excess glucose is not important; it could even be totally unintentional.

In fact, the body doesn't really care why its blood sugars are elevated: whether it is caused by over consumption of sugary foods, or whether it is caused by the over-eating of even healthy foods which contain carbohydrates. A person may not even be aware that the food being consumed has sugar in it.

The reality is that you can fool your friends, you can even fool yourself, *but you can never fool your body*. Our body will always react, sometimes in a positive way, sometimes in a negative way, but the reaction is always there whether we are aware of it or not.

Furthermore, if the diabetic is hyperglycemic for any length of time, this will cause damage; and if a diabetic remains hyperglycemic multiple times throughout his lifetime, the damage is multiplied.

We diabetics do not have the luxury to permit elevated blood sugars, regardless of the cause. The diabetic's body does not have the built-in defenses working at capacity to lower these dangerous blood sugar levels.

We don't have the necessary tools in our bodies to naturally reduce our blood sugar levels. This leaves us susceptible to all of the aforementioned complications. Without some type of help, we are defenseless in regard to blood sugar.

To recap: glucose levels rise due to an increase in the intake of sugars through consumption. This intake can be from sugary foods themselves, either in the form of sugar or any other type of carbohydrate, or they can also be from an excess of practically any food, even healthy foods. Now that we have learned about diabetes, the disease and its complications, what are we going to do about it?

CHAPTER THREE

MEDICAL TREATMENT

Hopefully the diabetic who finds out that there is a problem will go to a doctor for treatment. Let's take a look at some of the medical treatments available, and then we can focus more on preventive measures. The preventive measures are the keys that have kept me off my meds for over five years, and hopefully this will help you as well. However, it is paramount to first lower blood glucose levels, before we can attempt to prevent their increase.

The treatment for Type I diabetes is quite different than the treatments for Type II diabetes. As stated earlier, the main focus of this book is for Type II diabetics, but I would like to discuss some of the treatments for Type I.

The pancreas of the Type I diabetic is either producing less than 5 percent of the necessary amount of insulin, or none at all. This diabetic is therefore responsible to self-administer insulin in order to survive. Without insulin, the body cannot function. We need insulin to get the glucose into the cells to be converted in to energy. Also, without insulin, the glucose will "get stuck" in the bloodstream, and elevate to extremely high levels, causing a person to dehydrate, hyperventilate, and eventually fall into a coma if not treated, and die. This disease is called Diabetic Ketoacidosis (DKA).

On the other hand, if the diabetic self administers too much insulin, his blood sugar levels could decrease to an extremely dangerous level, resulting in shock and, if not treated, death.

It is therefore very tricky for a Type I to maintain regular sugar levels. It takes a lot of practice and education for the Type I to master the task of keeping the blood sugar levels within normal range.

The problem is that the body has this wonderful thermostat, a regulatory system, which keeps the sugar levels normal. However, the diabetic is lacking the insulin needed to maintain these normal levels, and therefore the thermostat system is useless. The diabetic basically has to mimic the pancreas, and become his or her own thermostat.

When blood sugar levels fluctuate, the diabetic needs to be aware of these changes and regulate the amount of insulin to administer. For this reason, Type I diabetics must check their blood sugar levels several times a day.

Type II diabetics however; do have insulin in the body. Their problem is more complex, and therefore the treatment is different. The problem is to get that insulin into the cells.

There has recently been an increasing trend by some doctors to begin treatment for a newly diagnosed diabetic with insulin shots as opposed to oral medication. There has been much success with this approach.

However, some diabetics still do better with the oral medications. There are many different oral anti-diabetic medications prescribed to try to help the sugar get into the cells, and newer ones are being produced as we speak. We will discuss just two for now.

One classification of drugs is the sulfonylureas. These drugs work by squeezing out of the pancreas as much insulin as possible and also by working on the receptor sites of the cells to accept the insulin transporting the glucose. These drugs however, can cause hypoglycemia due to the increase of insulin secretion. They also inhibit the production of glycogen in the liver, reducing the amount of stored glucose.

Another, more popular, drug used today is classified as biguanides. The popular Metformin (or Glucophage) is part of this class. The advantage with these drugs is that they don't typically cause hypoglycemia since they don't effect the insulin production at all.

Their primary focus is to affect the receptor sites in the cells. These drugs increase the binding factors of the cells to the insulin, so that the glucose can enter the cells and be used for energy. They also attack the liver by inhibiting the production of glycogen (gluconeogenesis), which also reduces the amount of stored glucose. Thus, this drug also has been found to help with weight loss, due to the decreased amount of glycogen (stored, converted glucose) in the liver.

In early stages of the treatment, these medications keep glucose levels from increasing, however, even with all this, if the diabetic does not make, *and maintain*, certain lifestyle changes, the disease will progress and oral medication will not suffice. The Type II will become like the Type I and need to take insulin shots as well as oral medication.

Among adults with diagnosed diabetes, 14 percent take insulin only, 13 percent take insulin and oral medication, 57 percent take oral medication only, and 16 percent do not take either insulin or oral medications.

What I had difficulty in understanding is, with all the modern science and medicine at our disposal, why can't we, as a nation, control diabetes? Not only can't we control diabetes, but also the disease is reaching epidemic levels. The incidence of pre-diabetics, those whose sugar levels are elevated (just not elevated enough to be considered a diabetic), has already reached epidemic levels. The fix to this public health crisis is simple: we just have to get the glucose out of people's bloodstreams and into their cells.

For the Type I, we inject them with insulin and it's done. Yes, it's a little tricky to imitate the workings of the pancreas, but it's definitely controllable.

Ironically, the truly difficult patient is the Type II. One would think that having naturally produced insulin is better than none. Yet, we see that Type II diabetics are dying at a much faster rate than Type I. Type II diabetics are losing limbs, having kidney failure and suffering from heart disease.

This is where modern medicine raises their hands and says, "We're doing the best we can. What else can we do?"

It is here that I believe that modern medicine is missing the boat. I do believe that in order to recover there is more that is needed than just taking some pills and or injections. There was something wrong with me, causing my sugars to elevate, and nobody could tell me what it was.

Once I had that light bulb experience that I spoke about in Chapter 1, I was able to control my diabetes. It is my belief that preventive measures in controlling diabetes is not just a theory, nor is it just another option for those who desire it. It is an absolute necessity for survival. I can't impress on the reader enough the severity of this concept.

There are more aspects to increased blood sugar levels than just the food we eat, or the lack of exercise. If we don't attack and treat *all* the underlying causes of increased blood glucose levels we will not be able to defeat diabetes. It's as simple as that; and this book will give you the necessary information to prevent *all* aspects of increased blood glucose levels, so that you may recover and live healthy with diabetes.

My wife works as an occupational therapist in a nursing home. The number of patients she sees with Type II diabetes with amputated limbs is scary. My heart goes out to these people whose lives have been ruined from this debilitating disease.

My wife tells me that these people (some as young as sixty and seventy years old) have given up on life. They are so depressed about their situation that they feel life is just not worth living anymore. It hurts me further knowing that there is a solution that could have prevented the amputations, and could have given them a fulfilling life.

Preventive medicine is not just an option or a nice idea; it is a must for the diabetic, as we will see in the following chapters. I'm not just talking about exercise and a healthy diet, there is an attitude about life that a diabetic must have if s/he wants to be healthy. The beauty of it is the rewards of living such a life have proven to me to be exhilarating. I play tennis several times a week, I travel, and I enjoy my kids and grandkids. I live life to the absolute fullest. The most important thing is that today I am happy. I am Awesome Al.

I would have never have been able to live this life with my elevated sugars. Taking nine pills a day and eating like a pig to satiate unbearable hunger, and just being absolutely miserable all the time. This was not a life. The worst thing was, unknown to me; I was killing myself, a very slow and painful death.

I have a choice today: to live and be happy, or die a diabetic death just as my aunt and grandfather did. The following chapters will give some practical solutions to live the happy, healthy life I have chosen, and which you too can choose.

CHAPTER FOUR

PRACTICAL MEASURES

The first step of my recovery was to accept the fact that I am diabetic, that diabetes kills, and that I must be willing to take certain actions to prevent the probable fatal consequences associated with diabetes.

We discussed earlier that retinopathy (eyes), nephropathy (kidney), and neuropathy (nerves), are the three main micro-vascular complications connected with diabetes.

Common medical treatments available for retinopathy include laser surgery, and vitrectomy. Vitrectomy is a procedure in which the surgeon removes a portion of the vitreous gel (thick, colorless gel that gives the eye its shape, by filling the large space behind the lens). This helps remove the floating blood vessels that are not able to clear up on their own.

These treatments are very successful in preserving a person's sight. In fact, even people with advanced retinopathy have a ninety percent chance of keeping their vision when they get treatment before the retina is too severely damaged. It is important to note that although these treatments are very successful, they do not cure diabetic retinopathy. Therefore, even after performing a successful procedure, the person may again develop complications if their diabetes is not brought under control.

The key to preventing blindness is early recognition and early treatment, before the retina is totally destroyed. It is therefore imperative for the diabetic to have an annual eye examination. Make sure to tell the ophthalmologist that you have diabetes, that way the appropriate eye tests will be performed.

For in between your annual visit I have included below an Amsler Grid. This is a self-test that everyone can perform in the privacy of his or her own home. The instructions are mentioned below, and ideally you should do this test once a week. It's easy and takes literally seconds to perform. This test is not only for diabetics, but also for anyone with a family history of macular degeneration.

In the test, the person looks with each eye separately at the small dot in the center of the grid, while covering the eye that is not being tested, and if one wears glasses, leave the glasses on during the test.

The Amsler Grid

Why Use the Amsler Grid?

It is important to detect a problem or change in vision at the earliest opportunity. The chance of saving eyesight is greater if detected early. Patients should be aware of what they are seeing with each eye. Treatment is no longer possible once the macula has been seriously damaged. Therefore, patients with early macular degeneration or with a family history of macular degeneration should test the vision in each eye, separately, at least weekly. The Amsler Grid is the best eye test to detect small changes in vision. *YOU SHOULD SEE YOUR EYE DOCTOR IMMEDIATELY IF YOU DETECT ANY CHANGES.*

Amsler Grid

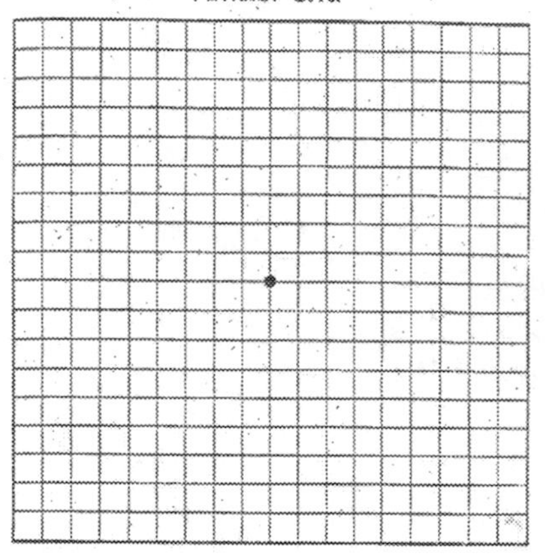

How to Use the Amsler Grid

1. Wear your reading glasses.
2. Cover one eye.
3. Look at the center dot and keep your vision on it at all times.
4. While looking directly at the center, and only the center, be sure that all the lines are straight and all the small squares are the same size.
5. If you should notice any area on the grid that appears distorted, blurred, discolored, or otherwise abnormal, please call your eye doctor right away.
6. Do this test for each eye.

Amsler Grid With Distortion

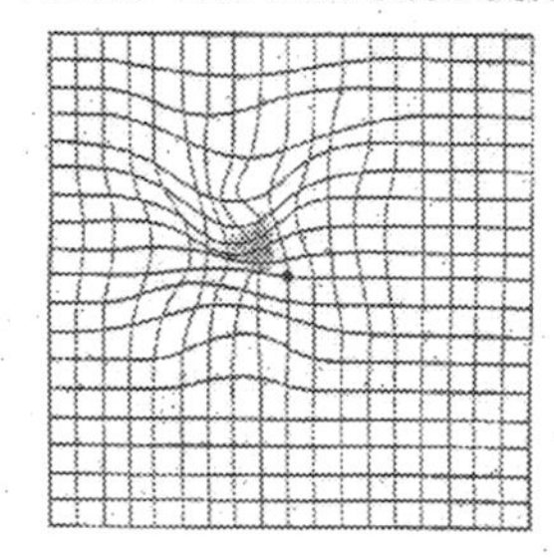

If this is how the grid looks to you, visit your eye Doctor immediately.

The main treatment for nephropathy, once proteinuria (protein in the urine) is established, is the use of ACE (Angiotensin-converting enzyme) inhibitors, which usually reduces proteinuria levels and slows but doesn't stop the progression of diabetic nephropathy.

These drugs are also used for high blood pressure and congestive heart failure by easing up the workload on the heart. This also helps for diabetics by reducing the risk of heart attack and stroke caused by macro-vascular diabetes. In addition, Ace inhibitors can help with other diabetic complications caused by retinopathy and neuropathy, such as eye damage and foot ulcers.

However, a side effect of these drugs is hypoglycemia (low blood sugar). Therefore, a diabetic needs to monitor his blood glucose carefully when taking these drugs.

The last and most severe micro-vascular complication is neuropathy. As was discussed earlier this affects the diabetic's nervous system due to decreased blood flow; which in turn affects wound healing, especially in the feet.

The feet are the furthest body-part from the heart. Therefore, it is logical that they have the most difficulty receiving blood. In a well-functioning body, the strength of the pumping heart as well as gravity makes it possible for the feet to be well nourished with the necessary blood. However, for the diabetic with neuropathy this task can be difficult. Furthermore, the (over) weight of the entire body rests upon the feet causing excess pressure, increasing the resistance to normal blood flow. Also the bottoms of the feet are rarely observed, leaving them susceptible to an unnoticed sore.

Restrictive clothing such as shoes, socks, stockings, and girdles, can be extremely detrimental by impeding circulation: these all need a looser fit. When buying shoes for instance, it is important to purchase them at the end of the day when your feet are tired and slightly swollen from the day. This will allow you to get bigger shoes that are comfortable and less restrictive, providing more room for your feet and toes. There are also specific shoes and socks made for diabetics. It is also advisable to rotate your shoes, and not wear the same shoes day in and day out.

Walking barefoot is a definite no-no. The loss of sensation at the bottom of the foot will prevent a diabetic from feeling a minor cut, which could become a major wound.

For this same reason, you need to be careful not to take an extremely hot bath, or leave a heating pad or an ice pack directly on your legs for any length of time. You won't be able to feel a minor burn to the skin that can lead to a major wound.

When cutting your toenails, it is advisable to go to a podiatrist to learn a proper technique such as cutting straight across the toe, and not tearing the skin, which could cause bleeding. Sitting cross-legged is another way to impede the blood flow to the legs, yoga practitioners beware!

Impeccable hygienic care is also extremely important. Washing your feet daily, then drying them well prior to donning any socks or foot-ware will prevent fungal growth that can lead to cracked skin. Check your feet daily, or if not, at least weekly, and notify your doctor if you recognize any discoloration of the skin or small wounds. Early recognition of problems can save that limb.

The aforementioned care is specific to certain parts of the body. To totally combat this disease we need to focus on the entire body. Neuropathy affects all blood circulation and most nerves, foot care and eye care alone even though important, just won't suffice. The best preventive measure for the diabetic is to reduce blood glucose levels and keep them normal.

Diet and exercise is always the topic of discussion in preventive care. "Eat less and move more," they say. Seems pretty simple, but is it?

As with any disease, diabetes has different stages. Furthermore, what's healthy for one person is not necessarily healthy for another. This concept is extremely important in the care of diabetes, especially when it comes to diet and exercise.

Typically food and exercise have opposite affects with regard to blood sugar levels. Food raises blood sugar, and exercise lowers blood sugar. However, for a person with elevated blood sugar levels, for example, in the range of three hundred or higher, "normal" exercise has the opposite effect; it will actually raise blood sugar levels.

Exercise produces stress in the body. Stress in the body triggers the excretion of cortisol, which in turn metabolises the glycogen stored in the liver and muscle tissue. This raises the blood sugar levels in the bloodstream. Alas, the diabetic is unable to process this extra blood sugar leaving an unhealthy elevation of blood sugar levels.

Therefore, for a diabetic with 300 plus blood sugars, mild exercise such as a fifteen minute walk, as opposed to a thirty minute run, three times a week, will help with blood circulation, but isn't strenuous enough to produce the stress leading to cortisol excretion and unwanted elevated blood sugar levels.

As one's numbers subside with medication and proper nutrition, more strenuous exercise is recommended. In fact, a diabetic (typically type I) may need to eat a snack prior to exercise to prevent a hypoglycemic episode as a result of the strenuous exercise.

Nutrition is the next topic, obviously an extremely important and an extremely individualized subject. (I have devoted the entire chapter seven to weight loss; however, there are some basic principles about nutrition that we will discuss first.) Cake, cookies, and candy are out of the question for us diabetics. They are just poison for us. Exception: for a diabetic (typically Type I) during a hypoglycemic crisis, such foods can be lifesavers.

Not only is the type and amount of food we eat important, but also the time of consumption is important. Generally speaking, eating after around seven PM is poison to the body. I must leave time for my digestive system to metabolize my food prior to sleeping. Since my metabolism has slowed down in the evening, the food I might eat too late at night just sits in my stomach turning to fat. (This is not the same for people who work a night shift)

Exception: a diabetic may need to have a late night carbohydrate snack at times to prevent a diabetic Somogyi effect or dawn phenomenon.

This is when the blood sugar is elevated in the morning for no apparent reason, either with or without a sudden hypoglycemic episode at around three AM. To prevent these phenomenons, there is an adjustment made to the evening insulin injection, and a late snack consisting of complex carbs are eaten.

There are three types of carbohydrates: sugars, starches and dietary fibers, all of which turn into sugar when metabolized, and hence raise the blood glucose levels. The only difference is in the amount of time it takes the body to metabolize that specific carbohydrate. Obviously sugar is the quickest, which therefore spikes the glucose levels the fastest when eaten. The glycemic index, which we will talk about, is a tool that is used to determine which type of carbohydrate spikes the blood glucose levels the quickest.

The diabetic must read labels when purchasing foods. When you look at the nutritional information be careful to read the "total carbohydrate": this gives an accurate calculation of the carbohydrate content in the food, which includes all three types of carbohydrates. Also, be aware that the information is per serving and not necessarily per package. Once again, to get the accurate calculation, you must read the serving size on the label.

As for sugars; a simple rule I go by is: if sugar, glucose, high fructose, honey, corn syrup or any sweet ingredient are in the first three ingredients, it's advisable to avoid that food. If they are in the fourth or fifth ingredient then it should be limited.

A lot of diabetics have a misconception when choosing to eat sugar-free foods. If the food is a carbohydrate such as sugar-free cookies, you're not getting a totally sugar-free food, since flour is a carbohydrate. Also fruit and fruit concentrates contain sugar.

Now about the glycemic index (GI). This is an index with certain guidelines to help you measure the amount of glucose in the foods you eat, as well as how quickly they spike blood sugars. The lower the GI, the healthier the food is for the diabetic, and vice versa.

A list of some of the high GI (seventy or more) foods is: white bread or bagel, white rice, popcorn, pretzels, corn flakes, and melons. Medium GI foods (55-69) consist of: brown rice, whole-wheat rye, pita bread, couscous, quick oats, and brown rice.

Some of the low GI, hence the healthiest (fifty-five or less) foods are: 100 percent stone ground whole wheat bread, rolled oats, corn, barley, bulgur, yams, legumes, and lentils.

Here is an example of some of the GI guidelines.

Lower GI	Higher GI
Fat and Fiber	Cooked or processed foods
Less ripe fruit or vegetables Whole Fruit	More ripe fruit or vegetables Fruit Juice
Whole baked potato	Mashed potato

However, the GI index is not recommended for early treatment of diabetes. Research shows that total carbohydrate counting, as well as the type of carbohydrate, is a better predictor of glucose intake than the GI. The GI is, however, recommended for fine-tuning a well-maintained diabetic.

Sounds confusing? It is. Nutrition is not an easy subject to tackle. For this reason it is highly recommended that you go to a nutritionist, and get on a healthy food plan. Eat more small frequent meals, rather than fewer large ones: this will keep the metabolism working, and don't eat at night unless recommended by your doctor or nutritionist. Fresh foods are always better than processed.

It takes time through trial and error to figure out what's good for you while still enjoying what you eat. Also, as your body changes so does your food plan. So go easy on yourself, persevere, but don't expect perfection.

The last subject in practical care is blood glucose monitoring. Monitoring your blood glucose levels is key to really determine if your diabetic treatment is working.

The best method is by taking a blood test called the Hemoglobin A1C test. This test is able to detect your sugar levels for the previous three months. It is recommended that diabetics take this test every six months. In between this test there is self-monitoring with a glucometer, an electronic device that tests a drop of blood, excreted from the tip of your finger. This test should be taken at least twice a day: once before breakfast, and then again around two hours after a meal.

The American Diabetes Association changes their desired recommended glucose levels periodically.

The most recent lab levels recommendation for the adult diabetic is as follows:

A1C	<7.0%
Pre-prandial plasma glucose (before a meal)	70–130 mg/dl
Postprandial plasma glucose (two hours after a meal)	<180 mg/dl
Random glucose (no specific time)	<200 mg/dl
LDL	<100 mg/dl
Triglycerides	<150 mg/dl
HDL	>40 mg/dl
Blood pressure	<130/80 mmHg

The ADA doesn't want blood glucose to exceed 200 at any given time. They want to keep the FBS (fasting blood sugar, taken first thing in the morning) between 70 and 130, and the glucose two hours after a meal below 180. The other levels are for blood pressure and cholesterol. As was explained; diabetes affects all systems in the body, and therefore, a healthy body in all aspects is necessary to control diabetes and prevent complications.

Until now we have discussed practical care for the diabetic, the different complications of this disease, as well as some of the remedies available to maintain a healthy blood glucose level. Even certain preventive measures were discussed, such as proper nutrition, eye and foot care, and glucose monitoring. This would all be academic if it wasn't a fact that diabetes is becoming an epidemic. There has to be something else out there available to help in preventing the onset, as well as the complications of this disease. It is true that genetics plays a major role in contracting diabetes, however, there seems to be a missing link in the equation: diabetes treatment plus self-care equals recovery.

This missing link was puzzling me. I believe that there is another aspect in preventive treatment that is absolutely necessary to defeat diabetes daily, and live healthy with diabetes. A discovery that I believe will permanently change the way we think about treating diabetes.

To answer this; let us discuss a particular circumstance when there are increased levels of glucose in the body and yet the insulin doesn't deliver the glucose to the cells, and that is in times of stress.

When a person is stressed, the adrenal glands (which we will talk about) release steroids. These chemical messengers from the brain prepare a person to either stand her ground or run away: commonly known as the fight or flight syndrome.

When a person is in combat and needs to stand and fight, or is in danger and needs to run away, her body reacts immediately to this situation. Her brain sends messages to the systems that are needed for this encounter to power up, and also sends messages to other systems that are not needed for the encounter to shut down in order to conserve energy.

When I'm in danger, I need to see my enemy, hence my pupils dilate (become enlarged). I need to retain fluid, so my kidneys slow down. I need alacrity, so my brain increases its concentration by receiving more blood from my heart. My arms and legs need to be fully powered up, so my heart sends more blood to these areas. I need more oxygen, so my respiratory system speeds up, my heart pumps faster in order to compensate for the increased demand for blood.

Stress requires and burns energy, sometimes, a lot of energy. Our bodies respond to various levels of stress in the same way it does to any dangerous situation. This energy comes from glucose. If there's no free glucose in our body, like after we've eaten and the food has been totally metabolized, the needed glucose must come from the glycogen, which is stored in the liver.

When the stress passes, the person calms down, and less energy is required. The message is reversed, the steroids are recalled, and insulin is released.

The excess glucose is absorbed, either through use by the cells or by transformation into glycogen to be stored in the liver, and all is well.

There is one more instance when steroids come out and raise blood glucose levels. To me, this was the eye-opener that gave me the incentive to write this book.

We mentioned earlier the adrenal glands. The adrenals are found on top of the kidneys. They are regulated by the hypothalamus, which is located in the center of the brain. I find the adrenal glands to be absolutely fascinating. A little more complex than the pancreas, which is a two-part thermostat, the adrenals are a three-part thermostat, also including the pituitary gland found in the brain. They have many functions; I'm not going to go into the entire purpose of the adrenals, just the one that pertains to this topic.

When a person is feeling down, this is actually a very subtle form of stress. I'm not even talking about depression, but rather that feeling that things are just not right, not quite being able to put a finger on it, and feeling that something is somehow, someway off.

I'm sure almost everybody can relate to these feelings. Such feelings can come from fear, anxiety, remorse, guilt, shame, doubt, and, most importantly, for my thesis: negativity. These bad feelings are caused by many factors and, if they continue, can lead to depression.

When these bad feelings arise, our awesome body, (in its effort order to uplift a person to homeostasis: a state of well-being), commands the adrenals to release a steroid called cortisol, a/k/a the stress hormone. This steroid, like the steroids released in the fight or flight syndrome, raises the level of blood glucose in the body since energy is needed to uplift the person's emotions. Then, when the stress has passed, and the person has calmed down, insulin is released and the glucose levels caused by cortisol are decreased.

Furthermore, cortisol not only raises blood sugars, but it also adds to abdominal fat (yet another cause of diabetes). As a diabetic gains abdominal fat the more depressed he gets from being overweight. The more depressed he gets, the more the adrenals release cortisol to calm him down to feel better. The more the cortisol is released the higher the blood sugar goes.

I was so troubled with this diabetic dilemma in my own life, not being able to get to the route of the problem in order to find a solution to my diabetes, that when I studied about these hormones in Nursing School I nearly fell of my chair. The answer to this whole diabetes problem as well as the obesity problem had been staring at us right in the eye all along. How could we be so blind? When I realized this, I *immediately* started to write this book. I said to myself, *"I must tell the world"*.

To recap in simple terms, when a person experiences trauma then a hormone called Cortisol (aka the stress hormone) is released, and the blood sugars increase. This trauma can come from stress, depression, anxiety, negative thinking, illness, or strenuous exercise. The body is affected regardless of the cause of the cortisol secretion.

Furthermore, Cortisol secretion causes abdominal growth (fat) which in turn causes diabetes. So for the diabetic, hypersecretion of cortisol is so detrimental that it can actually be fatal.

Furthermore, if a diabetic is eating a healthy diabetic diet and exercising, and is even taking medication to prevent high blood glucose levels, if the secretion of cortisol is not diminished than the diabetic will still experience high glucose levels.

Hence, for the diabetic, there is no difference between eating pure sugar or secretion of cortisol.

Simply, *Stress causes diabetes.*

You may ask; how can I prevent stress, stress happens? You are correct stress does happen, however, there are two types of stress.

There is stress that is traumatic to the body and is non-modifiable. Such occurrences happen in people's lives such as: loss of job, the deaf of a loved one, or getting ill.

These stressors are truly non-modifiable; however, the body in its brilliance uses Cortisol to keep the body in check.

Cortisol is a true friend when it is used as such and typically will not cause diabetes. It will raise blood glucose levels but that is transient.

The stress that is modifiable that can and will cause diabetes is the worry, the negativity, the self imposed anxiety, and the harboring over events that typically we have no control over. This will cause Cortisol to secrete at dangerous levels and thus become an enemy to the body. This is the stress we can control. This is the life saving changes we are talking about in preventive care for the diabetic. It's your choice, will Cortisol be your friend or your enemy.

Strange as it may seem, in the course of my writing I went researching in medical books and journals, and even though many state the fact that cortisol secretion causes hyperglycemia, I was unable to find any Doctor or published medical journal take this information to the next level, and discuss cortisol secretion as a necessary preventive treatment in the care for diabetics. This horrible cycle is self imposed. The body doesn't care if the increase in sugar levels is caused by sugar consumption, stress, anxiety, negativity, or self imposed trauma. Even if a person is taking his meds and eating a diabetic diet, his blood glucose levels cannot decrease without a complete prevention program. This is not a theory or a nice idea, it is absolutely necessary to combat this disease. In the following chapters we will discuss solutions tailor made for diabetic care, to *completely* prevent the elevation of blood glucose levels.

CHAPTER FIVE

The Source

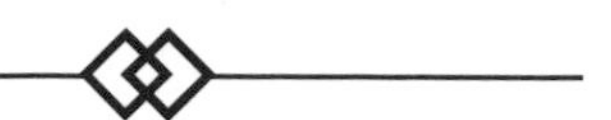

Diabetes is a horrible disease. It kills thousands of people each year. What's even scarier is that the available statistics are not very accurate. There are thousands, if not millions, of people walking around today who aren't even aware of the fact that they have this potentially fatal disease.

I was one of those people myself and nearly became a statistic. I was unaware of my condition for five years. However, once I did become aware and started my treatment, I fell into another oh so familiar category. I'll call it the Egypt syndrome.

In Egypt, there flows a great river it is called the Nile, or for our purposes called *De-nial*; yes, the old famous denial. What are we going to do about that?

It is my prayer that you will come out of denial and face the truth about your condition, and it is my hope to help you.

For me, the denial was caused by the lack of awareness of the disease and also that there is another solution other than medications.

I do believe, though, that this denial that I refer to is much deeper than simply a lack of awareness. I knew, for instance, that obesity was unhealthy. I would hear commercials about all the different ailments caused by obesity. The extra strain placed on the heart; that the heart works so much harder in order to pump blood to every excess pound of fat.

Furthermore, when I would go shopping in the supermarkets, I would see obese people who had difficulty walking. They were either in wheelchairs, or with walkers, many of them with oxygen tanks to help them breathe, sweating a lot, looking terribly uncomfortable. I would tell myself, "Oh that will never happen to me, I'm smarter than them."

Then I would glance into their shopping carts to see what they were buying–cigarettes. *What?! Cigarettes! Are these people insane!? Are they totally out of their minds!? Here, go buy a gun it's so much easier, and less expensive.*

Then I would notice the foods in their carts–cakes, nuts, chips, soda, deli meat, white rolls, etc. The cart was filled to the top with so much crap. Wasn't there even one healthy item in there?

What was wrong with them? Nooooo, that's not the question. You see, my cart was also filled with those same yummy foods. *What's wrong with me?! Yes me. Was I insane? Why couldn't I get it?*

All those ominous warnings, and I couldn't see that my bad habits, were just like theirs. It was like looking in the mirror when I saw what they were doing to their bodies. But, no, I didn't smoke, and I didn't need oxygen. But I could not (would not) see that I was killing myself in the exact same manner as they were. Why couldn't I understand that?

I didn't realize that not only was I physically killing myself with my bad eating habits, but also that the denial of my own situation was making the condition so much worse. I was focusing on them, anybody but me.

I became so judgmental, always judging everybody. There was something wrong with the way everybody else did something, and I was very glad to point it out to him or her. Well, wasn't that my job, to correct everybody else's mistakes? It took so much energy to fix the world that there was no time left for me to correct my own mistakes.

If the day came when I made a mistake and you told me, I became so defensive. I could never admit my mistakes. It was always somebody else's fault.

Then came the blame; I used to blame anything and anyone. I blamed my upbringing. That was easy and actually worked for a while.

However, when I got to be forty years old, with a wife and kids, going from job to job, blaming my childhood just didn't work anymore.

How long was I going to continue blaming events from twenty-five to thirty-five years prior as an excuse for my situation today? I blamed my wife, and then the bosses who fired me. Didn't anybody understand what I was going through? *"Nobody cares. They don't love me. I'll show them"*.

This inner frustration was killing me and I only had one solution to calm me. My only friend was food, and I would eat to suppress my feelings.

After a while this didn't work either. I would just get more frustrated at myself and then project that inner frustration at my loved ones. Yelling at them for anything and everything, feeling like crap all the time.

My despair, remorse, guilt, and shame, would always be followed by fear. I feared that it was never going to get better, and I was basically doomed. With all my talents, I had to concede that I was a born loser. I didn't just make mistakes; I truly believed that I was a mistake.

I actually believed this delusion for many years. Yes, delusional thinking. I have found this was not only the source of my troubles, but I am happy to say, delusional thinking has proven to be the start of my solution to diabetes.

I have lied to myself for so many years, that I'm pretty good at it. All those thoughts of uselessness have proven to be lies. I am *not* a loser, I am *not* a mistake, and I am *not* hopeless.

I can change. Life can be better, I can lose my weight, I can keep it off, I do look and feel great, I can control my diabetes, I can be happy today. Wow! Awesome stuff and I live that reality today and every day. This is my truth today, and it can be your truth, as well.

If you're still reading this book, you're probably asking yourself. *What the heck is he talking about, what does this have to do with diabetes and what do I have to actually do? How can I change my reality as well?*

Trust me, whatever your current situation, it can change for the better, and starting right now. Yes, not tomorrow, not Monday morning, but right now, at this very moment.

The first thing to realize is that it's *NOT YOUR FAULT. It's NOT YOUR FAULT. It's really NOT YOUR FAULT.* Say this to yourself a hundred times each day if you have to. *IT'S NOT MY FAULT, IT'S NOT MY FAULT, IT'S NOT MY FAULT, IT'S NOT MY FAULT, IT'S JUST NOT MY FAULT.*

Your current reality is based on yesterday's thinking. If you're anything like me, then you became aware, as I became aware, that my thinking sucked. It really did. So, if I'm not to blame, then where did this thinking come from?

Hold on, didn't I just say a couple of paragraphs ago that I had to stop blaming my childhood and everybody else for my mishaps?

Well, if I can't blame anybody else, and now I can't blame myself, than whom do I blame, and what exactly do I do?

Well I'm going to tell you another light bulb experience I had. I actually heard a similar comparison at a seminar I went to on child obesity, and would like to adapt the same concept for us.

Dr. David Katz, from Yale University, was using the analogy of a polar bear in the Sahara desert. All those layers of extra skin that keep the polar bear warm in the Arctic work against him if he would be in the hot Sahara desert.

We humans used to acquire food by hunting and gathering; this took a lot of energy and exercise. Once we did eat, we would consume extra food in order to store it for later; since we weren't sure when we would find food again. This type of eating did not cause obesity.

Today, there is such an abundance of processed foods available to us twenty-four hours a day. This food is easily accessible and can be prepared with little exertion. Our bodies naturally still store food for later, yet we don't use anywhere near the same energy acquiring and preparing the food. The human being is actually out of his natural habitat.

We are eating ourselves to death by consuming extremely large quantities of food, if not every day, then every weekend and holiday. We're not used to being surrounded by so much easily accessible food.

I am a creature of my surroundings. If I'm in the Arctic, I'm going to feel very cold. The simple reason is that I'm in a cold environment. If I'm in the Sahara desert I'm going to feel hot since I'm in a very hot environment.

Furthermore, not only am I living in a food-filled world, I'm also living in a very negative environment. Society, as I have become aware, and I don't really know why, loves negativity.

Some of the negative sayings I have heard over the years: the only guarantee in life is death and taxes, life wasn't meant to be easy, life just isn't fair, and the best one; nobody has everything.

These *opinions* have ruled my life and haunted me for years. That's right opinions. They are not facts; they are just somebody's opinion that I have taken on as a truth for myself.

When I am surrounded by negative talk, I become negative: not just in my attitude, but in my thinking as well. This negativity has been so ingrained in me that in order for me to have a positive outlook on life it has been truly a struggle.

I was recently standing in line at a concert, and a man was complaining to his friends about the uncomfortable weather the previous day. I could just see the bitterness on the man's face. He was just causing himself such anguish about trivial things that he couldn't control.

Now, how much control do you or I have on the weather, today or tomorrow? This was even better: it was about the weather *from yesterday*. What difference does it make today? Why get upset and take years off your life about stuff you can't control? I really felt bad for him and was just reminded of how vigilant I need to be in my positive thinking.

Another huge awareness I've had is regarding the media. I haven't listened to the news for over a year, and it is wonderful. The media has proven to be one of the major sources of negativity. It's just somebody's opinion about an event.

My wife had the news on recently and all I heard was: due to the recession this and due to the recession that: three times in one minute. I shut it off. No wonder there's a recession. The concept is shoved down our throats whether it's true or not.

The crazy thing is I used to love this stuff. I would rush to hear the headlines at the top of the hour, and would be constantly glued to the news. Then I would discuss it with my friends: "Hey, did you hear this terrible story on the news today?"

I became the messenger of bad news, as well. We would all stand there with those similar feelings of anguish, like the guy who was complaining about the weather. The usual comment was, after a huge sigh, "Oh well, what can you do, it's not in our hands anyways".

When somebody would ask me how I'm doing, it was also with that same sigh as well, and then I'd say, "Ok I guess." Even if I was a little happy, I would say, "Good, but..." That old familiar "but". No wonder I was Miserable Alan, living in such misery. I was not only surrounded by other negativity, but I would also self-talk myself into negativity.

Talk radio is another source of negativity I have found. I've also gladly stayed away from that. Those guys get paid to complain about anything and everything. What's more – it sells!!

I'm a diabetic. For me, listening to negativity is like eating a chocolate bar. Cortisol is released and the blood sugar just goes up; and the body doesn't care why the sugar goes up, the damage is done.

You may think I'm exaggerating. Let me challenge you to try for today to be aware of the negative thinking and talking that you're surrounded by. You may be pretty surprised at the extent to which this negativity surrounds you.

I am grateful to say that I have become so sensitive to negativity today; it rarely surrounds me anymore. When I sense it, I just move away and remove myself from the situation.

This negativity is so subtle, but it does exist and it permeates our every being. The more negativity I listen to, the more negative I become. The more negative I become, then the more negativity I attract.

The more I attract, the more I think negatively and feel negatively, and ultimately the more negative I become.

This horrible cycle went on for years and years. The stress level went up, my heart worked harder, cortisol was secreted, my sugars went up, and I spiraled into this horrible situation, of self-loathing, self-pity, and even thoughts of suicide. Sad but true, that hopeless lonely feeling of just wanting to give up returns, again and again. *Help! I'm sick of this. It isn't working.*

Congratulations. That is probably the best thing you could tell yourself. As I said in the first chapter, it was that pain that brought me to find another way.

Okay, you got me. Now what?

Starting from now, you are only going to think and say positive things about yourself. How do you go about it, if you're so used to the opposite?

I had the same dilemma, but I have a proven way to not only start to change for the better, but even when things get rough, to be able to turn things around to the positive. In the next chapter, we will start with some very basic tools that you can use right now. Get a pen and paper and let the fun begin.

CHAPTER SIX

THE PRACTICAL SOLUTION

Having read this far, you are already well on your way. Self-awareness is so important; it's actually 50 percent of the recovery process.

Until I not only knew, but also actually accepted the fact that I have a problem, I couldn't take care of it. Until I not only understood, but had also accepted the fact that I had a problem, I wasn't able to receive any help for myself.

The transformation from knowledge about the disease, to the release from denial, to accepting the reality that I have a disease does take time.

I wish I could predict a specific amount of time that it takes, but the truth is it's magical. It's nothing less than a miracle, and this miracle does take some time. That timeframe is different for everybody. For me it took about five years. Others get it almost immediately and some people live a lifetime and die without ever receiving the gift of reality.

I call it a gift because when I faced my fears and accepted my reality, I realized I had truly a beautiful life.

My mother always said, "Nothing is ever as terrible as we think it's going to be." For me, reality has become better than I could have ever imagined.

However, as was my case until I experienced some relief, I didn't believe this entire mumble jumble at all. I needed, not so much the happiness, but just some relief from the misery.

This release does take some work on your part and you can't wait for the feelings or the belief in the process to begin. In some ways it's a sort of catch 22. You won't feel better until you take some action, but aren't willing to take some action until you feel better.

You'll just have to rely on a little blind faith to begin, and watch out when you do because that relief will take place if it hasn't already. Now, let's take some practical actions to get some relief.

The first practical tool we are going to use is lying. Remember that I told you about delusional thinking back in Chapter 5. Delusional thinking is lying.

We're going to lie our way out of the misery of diabetes. I realized that I had lied to myself for years. I never believed I would get better. I never believed I would love myself. I never believed I would be healthy. These were all lies. The list goes on and on, and I'm sure you can add to this list some of your own.

Just for today, you are going to feel *awesome*. That's right, awesome. I don't care what is going on. I don't care if you don't have money to pay rent, if you don't have a job, if your sugar levels are elevated, or whatever your current reality is, it doesn't matter. Today is an awesome day.

Today say to yourself, I am awesome. Even if you don't believe it, when somebody asks you how you are doing just say *awesome* (even if you don't actually feel it). Just lie to yourself. It works. It really does.

At first it might feel strange. The mind may tell you: who are you kidding? You aren't awesome at all. You're a loser. You are hopeless. Why did you buy this book? It isn't going to work for you. Nothing has so far!

Don't pay any attention to that stinking thinking. They are not healthy, helpful lies.

I needed to tell myself that I wasn't going to listen to those negative lies. I was going to listen to the lie that I was feeling awesome.

The truth is that you really are awesome. You and I and every individual on the face of this earth are unique and each of us has a personal reason for being here that nobody else can fulfill. That's why you and I are here. God doesn't make junk.

There is a unique purpose for you, and nobody can take that away from you, not even you, and certainly not your thinking.

The missing link is getting *you* to believe the truth of your awesomeness.

My experience is that just by taking these actions everyday, by this self-talk, by this "lying" to myself, I actually began to feel awesome. Today, I don't have to lie anymore. I am awesome today; I actually feel my awesomeness today. What's even more beautiful is that I have also become a source of this joy to others.

When I tell somebody that I feel awesome, they lighten up a little too. What a gift. The strange thing is that that power has been instilled in me from birth. Every person, including you, has that same innate source of energy. Ironically, what I thought to be a lie is actually the truth and what I believed to be the truth has proven to be the lie.

The reason that this works is; that when I am telling myself something that is true, (even though I may not actually believe it) my inner self accepts that truth, I have inner peace, and life works.

However, when I lie to myself I lack inner peace and get frustrated, because unbeknownst to me my spiritual self can not and will not accept the lie. The frustration grows; and no matter how hard I try, life becomes increasingly more difficult.

The amazing thing is that with time I don't have to lie anymore. I actually feel the truth that I am awesome today.

Therefore, it is as clear as day that when I think I'm lying by saying I'm awesome, I'm actually telling the truth. In fact, it's probably the first time in my life that I'm not lying to myself.

What happened next was that I looked at my current reality, and it didn't coincide with this positive self-talk that I was saying. I realized that my current unhappy reality was a direct result of the negative self-imposed lies I had told myself for so many years.

In order to change my situation, I don't really need to lie. What I really need to do is tell the truth to myself. That real truth is that I'm awesome. The more I say this truth, the more I will believe it. The more I believe it, the more my reality has and will change for the better.

Once this happens I actually start feeling better. Amazing how it happens. I believe it's nothing less than a miracle.

This tool is something that anybody can start right now. Even if you're skeptical, try it: you may even like it.

My experience is that I really love it and actually look forward to the opportunity when I can tell somebody I'm feeling awesome. By saying this, I'm surrounding myself with more positive energy and that energy is flowing through to the point where I can actually feel the difference.

This positive energy helps me get healthy to an even greater degree than that damage which I received from the negative energy that I had filled myself with in the past.

I have learned to use another great tool when I'm feeling down. I close my eyes and visualize a place where I enjoy being, or a pleasurable event that I experienced. I need to do this for only seventeen seconds. I'm not sure why that amount of time works, but that's what I've been taught, and it has consistently worked for me.

Try this three times in succession. If you do this every day, in just three days you will start feeling like a different, happier person.

My friend who introduced me to this concept loves horses. She told me that she would visualize standing next to a horse, feeling the hair of the mane slapping across her face, running her hands across the horse's muscular body, feeling the wind flow through her hair. That scene would bring her such joy and pleasure.

For me, I love the beach. I visualize standing there wiggling my toes through the coarse sand, listening to the crash of the waves, and feeling the spray of the salty water on my face. I experience smelling that salty water and the seaweed in the ocean, and feeling the wind whip against my body and the warmth of the sun on my skin as I inhale the fresh air.

Wow! That feels so good. Just take it in and close your eyes and enjoy. Awesome. Do it now. I especially appreciate this visualization in the winter.

I've also been to some concerts. I stop and meditate on some of the songs I heard. I visualize the guitar solos and the drummer going wild. I even sing some of the songs myself, imagining being there at the concert. It brings me such joy. I'll go and listen to a music CD from that band and it just sends me right back to the concert. I can be happy for days from such a meditation.

If you don't have your own visualization, borrow one of mine. However, I'm pretty sure anybody can find some place they would love to be right now. The beautiful thing is that I can do this anywhere and anytime. Even if I'm driving, I can pull over to the side of the road and meditate. What a great tool.

These tools have proven to help me in desperate times as well as jumpstarting feeling good. I have found that when I'm feeling good, I gain some hope about my situation and life. I feel that this hope is imperative for me. It allows me to see life with a different perspective.

The real hope for me, which I pray will help the reader, is the realization that change is not just some fantasy, but is an actual reality. It can happen for you as well.

All those wonderful things that I have not only dreamed about, but also those that I thought I saw others possess, have become reality for me today. As much as I dreamed about them, deep down I believed that it was only fantasy. *Not going to happen to me* I would say. *Not in this lifetime*. Boy has that delusional thinking proven to be the furthest thing from the truth.

I wasn't able to believe that the positive life was possible for me until I experienced it. To experience the positive doesn't take a lot. It all boils down to attitude change and a change of heart. The amazing thing is everybody has the ability, the power to make that change.

This power, which I call spiritual in nature, is instilled in every human being. This being true, I don't need a huge effort to access this power at any time.

It has been actually in me since I was born, I was just never aware of it. In fact, I used it all the time. The problem was that I used my spiritual power to drive my negativity in response to my environment, instead of using this power to reinforce positive attitudes.

What does all this have to do with diabetes? Well, if you recall from chapter 2, I explained the vicious deteriorating cycle for the diabetic.

The need for glucose in the cell; and the cell not being able to get any no matter how hard the body tried, and the terrible hunger that was never satiated, which not only didn't help by eating more, it actually made things worse.

This caused weight gain, which led to depression, which both contributed to the increase in blood sugars from the secretion of cortisol.

To combat diabetes we must end this horrible cycle, and instead take the actions to cause a positive chain reaction for a healthy recovery.

I found that in order for this to happen, I needed some hope that it was possible for me. Once I had some hope, it became easier. I was able to start taking care of myself. I was willing to go to the doctor for treatment. I was willing to go the nutritionist to get a food plan. I was willing, to not only listen to the advice given to me by professionals, but was also able to put that advice into practice.

I don't use the words "able to put that advice into practice" lightly. I have found that my negativity actually caused a certain paralysis. As much as I heard the advice and the warnings, I couldn't bring myself to put these concepts into practice. I was powerless over taking certain actions. *Why, what's wrong with me? I know it's not easy to change certain behaviors, but why that feeling of hopelessness?*

Why the desire to give up when there is so much to live for? Why the complacency, the lack of interest to even try? So I failed a few times, does that give me the right to give up? I saw others try again, why couldn't I?

I see now that I had a mental paralysis. I believed the negative lie that "I just couldn't do it". I so completely believed this delusional thought of my inability to take action that I created for myself an actual physical paralysis. I really couldn't get out of the chair to seek help. I felt so lost.

That pain actually turned out to be a blessing. It was that pain that brought me to a place of willingness to change. I was willing to accept the reality of my disease and take care of it by making the proper choices. It was the only hope I had left since my present reality was so bad.

It was this hope that created an upward spiral toward a situation today in where I don't need my meds anymore. I would never have believed it possible at the time, but I knew I needed something different. My way certainly wasn't working, so I became, and still am, teachable.

Does that mean I'm cured? Unfortunately, no. I will live with this disease for the rest of my life.

At first that reality was painful because my situation seemed so grave. Today, I accept that reality with peace in my heart because I have found a solution. I have tools at my disposal today that allow me to live comfortably with diabetes.

Another interesting dilemma I came across. There were times when I became motivated; I would read a self-help book, a friend or relative would give me a kick in the pants, or a little talk or I would watch some TV show that would inspire me.

This would motivate me, and sometimes I would really give some effort to change. I found that after a short period of time, I would lose all interest. My old thinking would set in, shortly followed by my old behaviors. In fact, sometimes it would actually get worse than it was before I was inspired.

Why was this happening? Why couldn't I keep my commitments? It would probably be extremely interesting to analyze the reasons for this behavior. However, I really don't know how productive such an analysis would be.

This book is about taking action, and it has been proven to me that only through taking these actions have I been able to change my life for the better.

I heard an analogy about this once: when a train is coming and I'm on the track, it wouldn't help me much to analyze the reason for me being on the tracks. What would really save my life is simply to get off the tracks!

The same holds true for us. We can sit and analyze why we haven't accomplished what we wanted to. Why we've repeated the same mistakes over and over, why we're overweight, why we're so miserable, and we may even find some answers. However, what has proven to be the best medicine is simply to just take some action and move on.

But these actions need to be simple and attainable. If you set your goals too high, all you're really doing (and I have done this also many times) is setting yourself up for failure. You will not be able to accomplish those amazing expectations that you have set for yourself, and will therefore fail terribly.

I always came out of such an attempt saying, "See, I told you this wouldn't work. I don't even know why I try."

For this reason, I have used the word "today" many times in this book. This word has proven to be the key for me in all my accomplishments; today, today, today.

The two worst days of the week are yesterday and tomorrow. Yesterday and tomorrow are absolutely the two most impossible days to live in today. When you are feeling guilty for what you did or didn't do yesterday you can't function properly today. Yesterday is gone forever, and it will never return. Or, if you are worried about what's going to happen tomorrow, you will be absolutely miserable today. You can't predict the future, so what's the point worrying about it today.

Remember, you must live with diabetes. You truly want to do everything and anything in your power to live in good health. When you worry, you simply cause cortisol to be released in your body, your sugars elevate, and you're back to empowering you're diabetes, which degrades your quality of life. Don't go there.

You can't enjoy your life today when you are concerned about those other days. It is therefore of utmost importance that you live in today, just today. When you do this, life is so much easier.

Anybody can fight a battle for one day; it's those two eternities, yesterday and tomorrow that kill everybody. The only thing that you have the power to change is how you react to and live today.

The amazing thing is, when you focus on just today and make it the best day possible, you are actually changing your future life for the better as well.

Remember, your current reality is a byproduct of yesterday's thinking. Therefore, tomorrow's reality will be a byproduct of today's thinking. If today's thinking is awesome, there is a better chance for an awesome tomorrow.

How do you go about living today for today? Get rid of those guilty thoughts about yesterday which are crippling you today, and get rid of the fears of tomorrow and the hereafter which are paralyzing you today.

The first thing is to use the word "today". Many times I have worried about something for hours, and then realized it had nothing to do with today. It was either about remorse from yesterday or fears about stuff tomorrow. When I wake up in the morning, all I need to focus on is today. I set my plans for today and go about doing them.

During the course of the day, when those old bad thoughts creep in about yesterday and tomorrow, I remember that today I am awesome. Today and only today, I am Awesome Al. It's so simple and it really works. With time, it becomes a natural way of living.

Another extremely important concept is gratitude. An attitude of gratitude is priceless. When I fall into self-pity, remorse, or negativism, I cannot accomplish anything of positive value today. Gratitude has proven to be such a great tool to healthy living today.

My attitude of gratitude protects me from negativity, and gives me the strength to accomplish things I never thought possible. Whenever I'm feeling down for any reason, I quickly put together a gratitude list. The results are immediate: I feel better, I forget my misery, I move on to bigger and better things, I start to focus on the here and now, and I am able to do the next right thing.

The first time I heard this concept, my first reaction was: "I have nothing to be grateful for." Can you believe it? I must admit it did take me some time to master this "attitude of gratitude" thing. However, maybe I can help, so you need not suffer for many years like I did, because this stuff really works.

I don't know you and I don't know your situation, but whoever you are, and as bad as you may have had it (or believe that you have had it), you are here now, still reading my book, seeking a solution to your diabetes. This in itself is a reason for gratitude. Heck, just being alive is a reason for gratitude!

There are many people (and maybe you even know some) who have died very young, or who have died from some senseless killing, they aren't alive any more. Then there are people who are terminally ill, or are very sick right now. I really don't need to look far to have something to be grateful for.

Currently, you are reading a book about recovery from a fatal disease. You are seeking out ways to better your life. How many people do you personally know who would love to improve their situation? You are actually doing it right now.

Do you have food in your refrigerator? Is there running water in the pipes of your home? Is there electricity present in those wires? Don't take these things for granted; these are definitely things to be grateful for.

I was once turning off the filter of my pool since it had been running for twelve hours, and I didn't want it to overheat. I started to think about how many filters I have in my body. They have never shut down. It is absolutely amazing, not to mention awesome.

For the past forty-seven years, my heart has pumped blood at an average amount of five liters per minute, with an average rate of seventy-five beats per minute. Imagine that! Five liters a minute, that's two and one half coke bottles per minute.

What's more, my body's filters don't take a break. My kidneys filter my blood to excrete urine. My liver and spleen also filter my blood. The little hairs that line the inside of my nose and continue down my throat to my lungs called cilia; filter the air I breathe at an average rate of fifteen breaths per minute.

(These cilia by the way are destroyed by cigarette smoking, which then allow particles to get into the lungs, causing various diseases such as emphysema and lung cancer). These are just some of the major filters.

Every single cell has macrophages that engulf a foreign substance in the body, destroy it, and excrete it. Cells of every type have a lifespan. They die when they are used up and are recreated constantly. We don't even notice this happening because it's so subtle.

Scientists continue to discover new things about the body that they never knew before – not that they didn't exist, but they just weren't aware of it. There are so many different filters, cell divisions, cell deaths, reactions, absorptions, and changes in my body that are occurring at this very moment and so much more that nobody even knows about yet. Wow! This stuff is amazing and it never ceases to work while I'm alive, whether I believe it to be true or not. Are you grateful yet?

Imagine if one of these filters would shut down for a day or two, how about just an hour or two. The pain one would endure from not being able to go to the bathroom for instance would be devastating. Imagine if a cell died and the body didn't excrete it properly. The list of possibilities is endless. What a perfect machine we live in. You really don't need to look very far to find some gratitude.

Write down a list of one or two things for which you are grateful. Go crazy and make it five or ten, and then hold that list close to your heart, and say thank you. Thank you for everything in your life today. Thank you for the little things and the big things as well. Whatever your situation is, be grateful.

When you retire at night, go over your day and be grateful for a productive day. Go over the things that went well and be grateful. You can also look at the things that need improvement and say thank you. Yes, thank you for your challenges; for self-awareness is the key to growth. *Perfection is left for the angels, but growth is for humans and humans only.*

If I was perfect, I couldn't grow and become better. I need to be grateful for my mishaps as well. If it weren't for my pain, I wouldn't be helping you today. I am grateful today for all the pain and frustration I endured, it has brought me to a far better place than I could have ever imagined. I hope your gratitude list is growing by now.

Being grateful allows you to move forward, to accept your weaknesses, and improve your life. Gratitude will help you get off your chair, go visit the doctor, take his advice, and get healthy. You will be willing to go to the eye doctor for check-ups, check your blood sugars regularly, visit a nutritionist, start exercising, and get on with life.

If you do this with gratitude, with time you will hopefully have the same results as me. I am no longer on meds. Wow! My doctor took me off them more than five years ago.

This could never have happened if I was complaining all the time, I guarantee it. I would have never lost weight and I would probably be injecting myself with insulin today. I wouldn't be exercising and enjoying it. I certainly wouldn't be enjoying life and I wouldn't be Awesome Al.

Can it happen for you? Why not? It happened to me. Just follow the simple tools I have laid at your feet in the last two chapters. Try it for a week and see what happens. If you're honest with yourself you'll see some improvement and will want to continue.

My father, God bless him, is eighty-two years old and plays tennis three times a week. I said to myself, "If I wait until I'm eighty it won't happen" So, I started playing tennis again myself two years ago, and continue to play today and love it. I had given it up for so many years due to my weight and constant feelings of less than.

If you don't start today, it will just become harder tomorrow. Don't give up. It really works.

I believe I have been given another chance at life, a re-birth if you will. That chance is available for you as well if you wish; it can happen and will happen if you take the proper actions.

Think of the children's book 'The Little Engine That Could' telling himself, *I think I can, I think I can, I think I can.* Yes, you can. It is within your grasp. Grab hold of the rope and enjoy the ride of a lifetime.

CHAPTER SEVEN

WEIGHT LOSS

I would be doing you a disservice if I didn't mention weight loss. Even if you don't need to lose weight, good nutrition is imperative. Food is the primary source of glucose that the body needs for energy. Obesity is not a necessary criterion for contracting diabetes. There are many Type II diabetics that are not obese, as well as many obese people who are not diabetic.

Obesity has almost become an epidemic, and obesity definitely increases ones' risk of diabetes. Studies show that there are more people today dying from overeating than from hunger. This is the first time in the history of man that we have accomplished such a feat.

Does this mean that you need to be obese in order to catch diabetes, or that all diabetics are obese? Does this also mean that if you loose weight, you will be free from this disease? The answer strangely enough to all these questions is "no". There are many contributing factors to diabetes, and we will focus on some of them.

My mother, God bless her, said something very interesting to me. She said, "When I go to the doctor, he checks me over for just a few minutes, and then tries to diagnose my problem. I have been living with my body for seventy-eight years; don't you think I know my body the best?"

I agree with her completely. I was taught in nursing school, that what the patient says is correct. It is not my job to tell anybody how or what to feel. However, as a nurse, it's important for me to educate the patient, so that he or she can better understand what's actually going on with their disease. This helps the patient to actively participate in his or her own healing process.

For instance, when I was younger I was plagued with a potentially fatal skin disorder called cellulitis. I often had cracked skin due to athlete's foot. This allowed certain common bacteria to infest the outer layers of the skin on my legs. The bacteria caused an inflammation that easily spread if not treated with antibiotics. One time it got so bad that I ended up in the emergency room. Since my blood glucose was elevated (unbeknownst to me or my MD) my recovery time ran over more than the "normal" course of antibiotic treatment. The excess sugar in my blood was a great media for the bacteria to grow, and the reduction in blood circulation in my feet further retarded the healing process. Once I began to control my blood glucose, the celluiltis would clear up with the "normal" regimen of antibiotics. Understanding this dynamic has brought me to better health.

Now, let's take a little trip down Anatomy Lane. Let's try to understand what goes on in the body in relation to the absorption, production, and consumption of glucose (sugars). Isn't that the primary concern with diabetes, how to deal with sugar in the body?

The word *diabetes* itself comes from Greek meaning *sweet urine.* This is why we used to test for diabetes through the urine. Today, however, we test the blood giving us a more accurate reading of the glucose levels in the body.

I became aware through my nursing curriculum that our body is an absolutely perfect piece of machinery, engineered to work, not breakdown. This was a real eye-opener for me, especially since my primary conception of myself was that I was a failure. The different systems in the body work in complete, utter harmony, humming along in sublime perfection. It is imperative that a patient really understands this about his or her body.

Each human being is comprised of billions upon billions of cells combined together in perfection. Each cell contains DNA unique for that human being, and each cell has its own particular purpose within the body. Complete books have been written about the tasks and intricate workings of every cell.

Furthermore, our body is set up to not only function well while healthy, but is also able to protect itself from disease. The first line of defense is the skin, but our defense system in not just skin deep: it continues with the immune system. Soldiers (called T-cells, stored in the spleen) are sent to seek out and recognize any foreign objects in the body, and then come back and report their findings to the immune system planners.

If something harmful is detected, then killer cells are sent out to attack, destroy, and get rid of that dangerous, out of place particle. It does not belong in our perfect body.

Our body not only has a foreign body defense system, it also has an incredible repair shop to fix up trauma or harm to the body itself. It is a system that actually heals certain types of wounds, both internally and, on or just below the surface of the skin. The brain sends the messages and the extracellular matrix reacts. The body's repair system, that which heals our wounds, is mutilated by diabetes. That is why my cellulitis took so much longer to heal.

When I meditate on the intricate workings of the human body, I am overwhelmed by feelings of gratitude. What's even more profound is that each human being is born with all the necessary components to live a happy and abundant life.

When I took my nursing courses I found that although the body has it's own healing system, it is a primary goal of all health–care workers to not only help in the healing process, but also to try to identify hereditary as well as other factors that can cause defects and diseases. This early recognition of problems is a paramount principle in the preventive care of patients.

Having said all that, let's go a little deeper. Just like any machine, our body needs external help to operate and function successfully. A car needs gasoline as a source of energy and a battery as a catalyst to get it stated when you turn the key. Different fluids are needed to keep the car in running condition. There is engine oil to lubricate the pistons, transmission fluid for the gears, and power steering and brake fluid for the power assist. When a car has all its fluids and is well maintained, it will run well and last for years; hopefully far beyond the time the last car payment is made.

Our body is no different. We need fluid to lubricate our parts. We also need oxygen, vitamins, and electrolytes. The electrolytes include calcium, sodium, and potassium. These three minerals must always be within the normal ranges for the heart to beat, the blood to flow, the lungs to inhale and exhale, the brain to operate, the muscles to move, the body to function.

Just as a car needs gasoline to power the engine, we need a source of energy to power our body. The source of energy for our body is food and water. Without food and water a person will starve to death. A normal human cannot totally abstain from food and water for more than a few days. Alas, with too much food and water, we will also die before our time.

In the ordinary course of life, pre-mature death will come quicker for the obese person than the skinny person. We large people just don't tend to live as long as the thin ones. Just go to a nursing home. It is hard to find a really old, obese person. All the ninety year olds are skinny.

The same holds true with abnormal blood sugar. The hypoglycemic (low blood sugar) person is at a greater risk of dying younger, with a much more rapid decline in their health status, than the hyperglycemic (high blood sugar) person.

A person can live for years without even realizing that they are hyperglycemic. The average person finds out only by chance that they have diabetes, and typically, when they do find out, they have already had it for five to ten years.

This was true with me, as I related in the first chapter. I only found out by chance that I was diabetic, because I needed to take a blood test to drive for a taxi service. My blood sugar (blood glucose) was very elevated: three hundred thirty-two. The doctor told me that I had had diabetes for at least five years, and that damage to my kidneys had already begun to take place. My kidneys were already secreting protein into my urine, a classic symptom of diabetes. I was only thirty-five years old *sigh*.

When a person ingests food, the digestive system – starting in the mouth – breaks down the food through chewing, that is, for those of us who still bother to chew. (How I used to just gulp huge chunks of food in my craziness.) As the chewed-up food passes down the esophagus and through the stomach and intestines, it is further broken down and gradually gets metabolized into different nutrients, vitamins, proteins, glucose and waste.

The nutrients, vitamins, protein, and glucose are transported via the bloodstream to the various body systems that need those particular chemicals.

Our various bodily systems and functions have specific needs that require the specific bit of food that we have consumed and metabolized. So long as our body is functioning in a healthy way it "knows" how to distribute right nutrients, vitamins, protein, and glucose and we don't have to consciously figure this out. Just as in a car, the competent mechanic doesn't put anti-freeze into the brake lines, or transmission fluid into the radiator.

Normally, people know how to eat in ways that they know to be healthy, and our bodies take care of the rest. But I'm not so normal, I didn't know how to eat healthy, that's why my Doctor had to order me to go to a nutritionist. One of the consequences of over-eating is that we can accumulate excess nutrients, vitamins, protein, and glucose.

When there is more glucose in the body than is needed for that moment, the body stores the excess glucose in the liver (the body's storage tank). This glucose is stored in the form of glycogen, and when more energy is needed, the liver transforms the glycogen back into glucose, which is then transported to the cells for use. When the liver-tank is full, the excess glucose is converted into fat, and is stored in fat cells throughout the body, primarily in the abdomen. Any food eaten in excess, even "healthy food", will eventually turn into glucose and then fat.

People lose weight by ingesting fewer calories than the body needs to function. The body, which needs to get energy from somewhere to function, has no choice but to turn to its storehouses of fat, and transform that fat back into glucose, thus there is less fat in the body and weight loss occurs.

This common knowledge has seemingly not helped society. Obesity has become an epidemic and it is also a major cause of Type II diabetes.

In recent years, obesity among adults has risen significantly in the United States. The latest data from the National Center for Health Statistics show that 30 percent of US adults twenty years of age or older (60 million persons) are obese.

If you're not sure whether you are obese or not, there is a simple calculation for you to figure it out, this is called the BMI (body mass index). This is a simple calculation, which measures the percentage of body fat in your body.

First measure your height in inches and your weight in pounds. Then multiply your height by itself (squared). Divide your weight by the result of your height squared, and then multiply that number by 703.

The equation should look like this: weight in pounds\ (height in inches x height in inches) = "a number". Take that number and multiply it by 703. This number will be in percentage for, which is your BMI.

Example: weight 150 lbs, height 5'5" (65 inches)
65 x 65 = 4225
150/4225 = 0.355
0.355 x 703 = 24.96
Explanation of results:

Below 18.5	Underweight
18.5 – 24.9	Normal
25.0 – 29.9	Overweight
30.0 and above	Obese

As was previously explained, obesity blocks the flow of insulin deliveries into the cells. Furthermore, a recent study from the Ben-Gurion University in Israel suggests that typically cells communicate with other cells. This communication is necessary to secrete compounds to other cells and to organs such as the liver, pancreas, and the brain for optimum health. The adipose or fatty tissue, specifically in the abdomen, becomes dysfunctional and actually mis-communicates with other cells. They become a source for common diseases attributed to obesity, like Type II diabetes and heart disease.

In simple language: fat cells (specifically) in the abdomen send distorted messages to the liver and pancreas. This in turn distorts the thermostat-system, which leads to irregular secretion of insulin by the pancreas, and irregular secretion of glycogen by the liver; both of which cause diabetes.

This study has added to the body of proof that obesity is a major cause of diabetes.

Leading an obese life style is a poor plan for everybody and is even more destructive for the diabetic. There is no question that being overweight is troublesome for anybody, but for the diabetic being overweight just complicates things further.

With all this awareness, as well as the fact that the American people spend so much money on diets, why is obesity still increasing worldwide? Why is it so difficult to lose weight?

There are many studies and books written on this subject, and I'm not here to regurgitate or repeat what is already known. I just want to share my experience with obesity and weight loss, and what worked for me. I've got credentials; I have been able to maintain a 100 lb. weight loss for over five years.

I don't believe there is one single solution that will work for everybody, since every person is different. Therefore, the food plan (not diet) that works for me is not the same food plan that may work for you. There are some people who can tolerate certain foods or combinations of foods. Yet, there are other folks who have extreme difficulty with those same foods. Every person's metabolism works differently as well.

Having said that, it would be foolish of me to provide food choices as advice to you to help you with your weight loss. Your individual food plan is the job of a nutritionist, working with you, on a one-to-one basis.

However, there are some general underlying causes that promote overeating and the awareness of these characteristics has proven to be beneficial to me.

The first simple question is: Why would any person do something to himself that is so detrimental on a daily basis? Why would an individual not only eat the wrong foods at the wrong times, but also eat enormous portions that were far beyond their needs for survival?

The consequence of one's overeating and poor food choices can really harm them. I'm not just talking about the after effects of a heavy meal, like heartburn, I'm also not just talking about the health problems that come from poor eating, like diabetes, high cholesterol, and other harmful consequences.

I'm talking about those horrible feelings the next morning, the throwing up from over-eating, the stomach aches, the bloat ness, the difficulty sleeping, the difficulty breathing, not to mention the embarrassment of being fat. The clothes that never fit right and the effort it takes to find right fitting clothes.

The not being able to bend down to tie our shoe laces, the hardships we have getting out of a chair, and the difficulty getting into and out of a car, the tight feeling of sitting on a plane, on a bus, a taxi, or in a theater, or trying to get to our seat. The emotional stress it causes, feeling people are always looking at us, embarrassing us, and making fun of us.

At parties, I was always hanging around the food. And those buffets, oh my God, I thought I died and went to heaven. The horrible expense of buying all that food, it was just never enough. Yet those buffets and horrible eating habits are killing us. Why would anybody in their right mind do this to themselves? It's absolute insanity.

Sure there were days when I didn't overeat, but they were few and far apart. I mean, I don't put my hand in the fire every day, so why did I overeat almost every day. For me overeating was definitely painful, yet I wasn't able to stop. I have tried many diets since I was thirteen years old. I got so desperate that I even did something I swore I would never do - take diet pills. Nonetheless, all these attempts turned out to be vain, since the day ultimately came when something happened and I ate again. What was wrong with me?

I have tried so hard to answer these questions, and through my recovery with diabetes have found some practical solutions that really work.

So, in reality, we're dealing with two issues here, the first: weight loss, losing those extra pounds of fat that are killing us. The second issue, which was even harder for me to deal with, is keeping the weight off.

How many times did I lose the weight and then ended up gaining it back again, and more? I had already found a solution to overeating, so why would I go back to overeating again?

I mean if you really think about it, it feels so much better to be skinny. I can breathe better, move better, and can climb the stairs easier; why would I go back to killing myself slowly with overeating? This just blows my mind. Help! What's wrong with me?

To quote Dr Katz again from Yale University, "It's not our fault, it's just not our fault". There are 3900 calories of food per person, manufactured in America each day; this is double or more the average daily requirement for an adult. The companies market these products in various fashions, and we are lost in a jungle of food. Yes, man was made to live in a jungle, but not a jungle of food.

Some of the fast food joints are opened till 1 AM, or later. I don't think there is a more detrimental action that one can do to their body than eat at night, and not just any food, but fatty fried foods at midnight. The metabolism has slowed down for the night, and all that food is just turning into fat, since it's not getting metabolized.

So once again this environment we live in is making it difficult for us. Now, what are we supposed to do about it? There has to be a way out.

Let's first focus on weight loss. No question about it - obesity is a problem not only the United States, but also worldwide. Yet, Americans spend billions of dollars each year on diets and weight loss treatments. So again why do we have such a problem with eating healthy? The solution is definitely out there, so why are we missing the boat?

If you're anything like me, just the thought of losing weight is absolutely terrifying. How will I live without my stash? I don't actually need to eat the crap everyday; I just need to know it was available for me when I want it. When told to control my portions, I thought I was going to die. "You want me to eat only that tiny portion, how will I survive?"

I mean really, only one portion, and look at the size of that portion; I'll never be able to survive on that.

Then I would eat it, and watch my clock until my next food would be due. When it did finally come, I thought: this is not enough and what and when am I going to eat next? After doing this for a few days, I would say "to heck with this" and just go binge. I was so happy when I took those first lustful bites. Actually, the excitement of going out to buy my food was enough to make me feel better without even the eating.

I was so obsessed with my food that I never really ate it. I just shoved it down my throat. No wonder I never felt satiated or satisfied. The transitory good feeling of eating whatever I wanted, whenever I wanted was short lived; it didn't take long for feelings of worthlessness, self-pity and remorse to set in.

Oh, no need to worry, I had a solution for those feelings as well. Yep, you guessed it, eat more. That cycle continued over and over again, until I had built up a pretty good record of failure. I was the king of failure when it came to weight loss.

Another interesting trigger for my failure was the scale. It has proven to be almost as annoying as eating cake while trying to lose weight. I would work really hard on my diet, and then I would go on the scale. One of three results would occur: weight loss, weight gain, or no change.

If I didn't lose any weight, after "all that work", I often felt disappointed and Miserable Alan. My solution for feeling miserable was to eat more food.

If I gained weight: *well forget it, this diet isn't working, so to hell with dieting.* As a side note, if I gained weight while dieting, I certainly wasn't following the diet too well, but I would never admit that. God forbid.

Strangely enough, when I lost weight, I would feel good. Ironically, I then felt I was entitled to eat, as I really wanted, since I was skinnier, even if I had only lost 2 or 3 pounds. So, it didn't matter the number on the scale, I always ended up eating more food.

This must certainly be just another example of my insanity. I was just as much a slave to weight loss as I was to overeating. I couldn't see a way out whatever I tried didn't work. I was a failure, I was hopeless, and I was a mistake. These core beliefs haunted me for so many years.

My way wasn't working, and I needed a way out. No wonder I was suicidal, it was the only solution that made any sense and it was the only solution I hadn't tried. I am grateful to my guardian angel that I was saved from this calamity.

Yes, suicide is a calamity, and it doesn't help anyone. There is another way out. I didn't believe it at the time of my despair. I would have missed out on so much life filled with purpose, fun, and happiness had I taken that route of ultimate selfishness.

My experience has shown me that once again attitude plays a major role; both in weight loss and weight maintenance. I knew my relationship with food wasn't good, so how was I going to change that?

The first light-bulb experience I had: food wasn't making me happy anymore. I had used food to numb my feelings; it was my best friend. When my fears and discomforts were still present even after I ate, I had no choice but to take an honest look at what I was doing. *Food doesn't work anymore*.

It just wasn't working anymore, not only didn't it make me feel happy; it actually made me feel miserable. Since it didn't cover up the feelings anymore, I had an added despair after overeating. I was left with two discomforts: first, being the unhappy reason that brought on the overeating binge, and second, feeling crappy for overeating again.

However, overeating was the only thing I knew to make me feel good. Food had ultimately failed me terribly. I was between a rock and a hard place. I couldn't eat because it made me feel horrible, and I also couldn't *not* eat because it was the only thing I knew to make me feel good.

The first thing I became aware of was that I was confused, not just with food, but with a much deeper concept: pleasure and happiness. Pleasure and happiness are not the same; I thought they were.

Pleasure is taking some external object and using it for physical enjoyment. It could be a new car, a new house, even a tasty food. It could also be a relationship with a significant other, a spouse, a friend, or a family member. It could be a vacation, a swim on a hot day, even a huge salary raise at work. All these externals can bring pleasure.

However, the pleasures of these things always wear off and a new external object is needed to feel pleasure. The reason for this is because physical pleasure is limited by nature, and can therefore only give limited amounts of pleasure. Pleasure doesn't have the power to bring happiness.

Happiness, however, is spiritual in nature. It is a deeper feeling that not only lasts much longer, but also feels different. It feels different and a lot better than pleasure.

Ask yourself; how many times did you say "if I only had this" or "if I only had that" (especially with regard to food) I would be happy? Think: when you got it: were you happy? Are you happy now even though you received this desire of yours?

My experience has been that when I did receive whatever it was I was wishing for, the happiness was short lived; and soon I wasn't any happier than I was before I got it. The truth of the matter is I didn't feel happy at all. I felt pleasure; which, by the way, was exactly what I was supposed to feel since this physical object was only capable of doing that, giving pleasure.

Happiness doesn't need any externals; it is spiritual in nature and therefore is found deep with in me. I have the capacity to be happy, no matter what is happening around me. In fact, I don't need to change anything at all in my life, absolutely nothing, and I can be happy right now. I just need to tap into that spiritual source within me, and I can be happy.

I'm not talking about God, or any religious concept. Spirituality is a real energy that we all have.

Just the fact that our hearts beat, and our lungs breathe, is a proof that each and every one of us is a spiritual being. I believe that the difference between a corpse and a living person is that spiritual source which resides in each and every one of us.

You may ask, what does this have to do with weight loss?

Well, quite a lot actually. Most of my eating, I have become aware, was emotional in nature. When I was excited or anxious, I felt hungry. Especially when I was nervous or afraid, I thought I was starving. This could happen at any time, but especially at night. For me, I was afraid, (sub-consciously) that I just wouldn't last the night without food. I had eaten dinner already, and the next meal wasn't until morning. Or, I was just nervous about something that was going on the next day, or something that happened during that day.

Regardless of the reason, I felt an emotional hunger that wasn't physical in nature at all. This is another example of the lies I told myself.

Today, I eat dinner usually no later than six, and I don't eat anything until the next morning, and I feel great. I'm not run down, I actually have more energy, and I'm not hungry. In fact, some mornings I power walk a couple of miles on the treadmill. Before breakfast!

I've realized that the only time I feel any hunger at night is when I'm nervous about something. It's never physical hunger. I surprised myself by learning that I didn't actually die after twelve plus hours without food. Go figure.

In order to not overeat today, I have to be at peace with myself. I am talking about an inner happiness, or better yet an inner peace. When I don't feel that inner turmoil of excitement or frustration and I'm at peace with myself, I don't need any externals, not even food, to make me feel good. I am a complete human being, running on the energy instilled in me. The calm and peace that I feel is so wonderful. I am not anxious or sad. I'm not nervous or excited. I'm at a perfect calm. It's like a cloud of serenity has engulfed me, and I'm just okay.

Everything is wonderful and I'm at perfect harmony with the universe and myself. I have become aware of all my surroundings and myself. I have a real knowledge of who I am and my place in the world. I appreciate nature. I hear the birds chirping, the wind howling, and the presence of the trees and the grass. Life is wonderful. I am living in the present, and it is by no coincidence that it is called the present, since the present is a real gift.

Once you experience this, there is truly no equal. It is absolutely amazing and it is the way I live today and have lived this way for the past few years.

When I live like this, everything takes on its true identity, including food. Food is no longer a source of desire or an escape; it is merely a substance that I use for my sustenance. I need food as much as I need water and air. I don't over breathe, I don't over drink, and I don't need to overeat either. This is the attitude change that is so important to weight loss. I don't need to overeat to douse my problems or become happy.

The awareness of my misconceptions about food also really helped me. I had deluded myself for years that food was my friend. I abused food; it became a poison that turned against me. It's curious how things happen like that.

The antidote to that poison; my recovery was to use the same tactic that had destroyed me – to allow food to help me. I had lied to myself for years that there wasn't enough food for me. I had to lie to myself that what I *was* eating *was* enough. Delusional thinking becomes my savior.

You know what, my healthy food plan really is enough, and the proof is I'm still alive. Granted, at the beginning I was hungry, but that only lasted a few days. I haven't felt real hunger in a long time.

Another truth I must tell myself is that I can lose weight and get healthy. Not only am I capable of losing weight, but also I am worthy of losing weight and being skinny. I am a child of God, and have as much right to be here on this earth as anybody else. I must tell myself this constantly, because those old fears can easily creep in. It's just stuff that I've told myself for so long, I must start telling myself new stuff that is really true. I had to stop the negative self-talk; it was killing me.

This really works; and it must start today, not Monday morning, not tomorrow, but today. Today, you can say that you're going to eat healthy, and you're going to make good choices, today.

When those insane thoughts of eating the wrong foods come in, just say: "I choose not to eat those foods, today." Just for today you can choose to eat healthy; tomorrow you can choose to be insane and eat unhealthy. The one day at a time approach, the just today I'll make the healthy choice takes away the fear of "never ever". The "never ever" thought can defeat anybodies resolve. I have no power to live healthy today while I'm caught up thinking about the rest of my life.

When you get a craving for a certain food, you can do the same thing by saying to yourself, "I'll have it tomorrow."

The interesting thing about cravings is that whether you indulge in them or not, within a few moments the craving subsides.

Amazing! I thought all along I was going to die if I didn't eat the food right now. I found out that it doesn't matter whether I eat the stuff or not. The food itself doesn't quiet the desire, time does. The food is not the solution there is another solution: time.

My skinny brother used to say: "just because it's there in front of you, doesn't mean you have to eat it". I never understood those words until recently. How could I have been so wrong, so may times, for so many years?

Well by now you are probably well on the way to weight loss, so how are you going to keep it off?

The truth of the matter is the remedy is not out there. It's instilled in each and every obese person. You don't need anything or anybody else to lose weight and keep it off.

You have the ability to lose weight and keep it off. Tell this to yourself constantly if not daily, until you actually believe it. Yes, delusional thinking again. I did it, so can you.

The same effort that you exerted to gain weight can be used to lose it and keep it off. All that is needed is a change of attitude.

For myself, I needed to realize that I did not get to 310 lbs from one slice of pizza. It took years of terrible eating habits for me to gain all that weight. It is only natural that I wasn't going to lose my weight or change my habits in one day.

It takes time and patience. However, if you don't start today, it won't ever happen. The other thing is that it's not a race, and there are no deadlines.

Furthermore, even after you lose weight those old fears may creep in. The fears that this will never work; or that you'll never lose weight, or what's the point in trying anyways, you're just going to gain it back?

This is the reason that diets never worked for me on a long-term basis. I set myself up for failure before I even started. I actually caused the diets to not work (subconsciously, of course) by not believing in myself. That self-doubt is such a killer. I actually couldn't wait to get to my goal weight so I could start eating like a pig again.

Even after losing a tremendous amount of weight, I gained it back. I would look in the mirror, and not recognize myself; it was as if somebody had placed my head on a foreign body. *I couldn't think skinny.* I was so relieved when I gained my weight back because that was the person I knew. It's insane, but that was me.

In order to live a skinny life, you need to have a skinny mind, no matter what size or shape your body is in.

When I was fat, I lived a fat life. I had a fat brain, I thought, talked, and acted like a fat person. Even during and after weight loss, I still had the brain of a fat person.

Let me give you some examples to help differentiate between fat thinking and skinny thinking.

If you said to a skinny person: "Wow, you're so skinny. You must never eat." Nine times out of ten they will say: "What do you mean? I eat a lot".

Now, go to a fat person and listen to what they say. "Me? I haven't eaten all day," or "I barely ate anything at the party yesterday." Obviously something is wrong here. If the skinny person ate a lot, that person would be fat. If the fat person didn't eat all day or very little, that person would be skinny.

Now just to prove my point a little more; go to a buffet or a cafeteria where people fill their plates and then pay at the end. Look at the difference between the plates of the skinny and fat people. You will be amazed as I was when I tried this.

Skinny people are skinny because they don't eat a lot. Fat people are fat because fat people overeat. It's as simple as that.

When I accepted this fact, I started to lose weight. When I stopped focusing on the weight loss, and what I could or couldn't eat, but started to believe in myself that I could do it, the weight came off and stayed off.

I also had to stop using the word diet and start saying I was on a food plan. A food plan that I could live with for the rest of my life.

The difference is that a diet for me means: "*die yet*?" It means deprivation and starvation and doing without. That will never work, not for me, not for anybody.

A food plan, on the other hand, is the abundance of nutrients you are give your body so you have the necessary energy to live an awesome day. You must eat to live, and eat you shall. Eat healthy, good, nutritional, and tasty food.

Your body will be happy when you eat, and you will be happy to treat yourself like a king. You will be satisfied when you finish, and won't feel stuffed or deprived. What a beautiful thing God has given us called food.

With such an attitude toward food and eating, you can lose any amount of weight, and keep it off for a lifetime. It is an attitude for today. Yes, just for today. Nobody loses weight worrying about tomorrow, but you can definitely loose weight and keep it off today.

CHAPTER EIGHT

Long Term

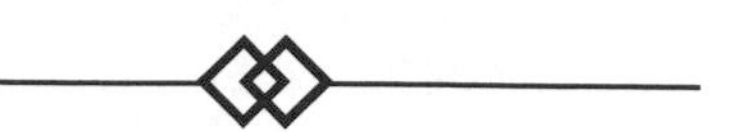

Congratulations, you've made it. If you are reading this chapter, then you have already begun to feel positive changes in your life. If you haven't experienced any differences yet, then go back and reread chapters 4 and 5. The solutions are there for you; they just need to be brought into practice.

There is a deeper aspect of my recovery that I struggled with, and I have noticed the same struggle in others. Once I started to feel better, I became complacent in my recovery. I began to feel that I had beat diabetes. I didn't recognize the reason I was feeling better and was off my meds; I didn't appreciate that my daily meditations of gratitude, that my diligence with my food plan, and that my exercise regime were all truly the reasons for the daily reprieve I was having from my diabetes.

I would forget for a day that I have a disease called diabetes. My mind would tell me that I could do the fun things other people are doing and that I could eat like other people without suffering the familiar or, even worse, the foreseeable consequences.

I once started to be more lenient with my food plan and, for instance, started eating "sugar free" foods while studying. This is such a huge mistake.

Yes, it is not actually sugar, but the sugar alcohols contained in sugar substitutes are also poison for a diabetic. Also sugar free cookies are full of carbohydrates that quickly turn into glucose once digested. The "sugar free" chocolates are just another misconception, loaded as they are with sugar alcohols that it's just like pure sugar itself. In fact, the ADA considers 2 grams of sugar alcohol to be equivalent to 1 gram of sugar. ` My body's chemistry was not fooled, and that horrible cycle of gaining weight, elevated blood sugars, feeling remorseful for eating the wrong foods, which causes the secretion of cortisol, which spiked my blood sugars started again and before I knew it, I was back to the races, feeling worthless and eating everything in sight, due to the unsatisfied hunger caused by my diabetes.

For me, I must remember *daily* that I am a diabetic, and therefore must follow a certain diabetic-safe lifestyle. This doesn't mean I need to deprive myself, but I must behave and think in ways that a non-diabetic doesn't. The day I forget that I am a diabetic is the day I'm in trouble. It won't take me long to spiral back into big trouble even if I'm not taking any medication for diabetes. The delusion that I have eradicated diabetes must be broken. Diabetes cannot be cured, but it can be controlled.

Another very interesting discovery I had, as I became healthier, was that when I started to feel better, I became very bold.

I started to go after things that I thought I wanted to do, like finally become successful, without prior investigation, about my motives, going off half-cocked, so to say.

About the time that I was doing much better with my diabetes, I was working at a bagel store that was really taking off. My boss and I discussed all aspects of his operation, and I truly thought I had what it took to be able to mirror the success he was having. With his blessings I opened a bagel store in a neighboring community thinking this was the way for me to become successful. I didn't open the bagel store because I wanted to run a bagel store. I opened it because I wanted to be successful. Let me tell you, I didn't make it. Not only was I not successful, but so much worse for my family and me: I lost a fortune in this endeavor. Remarkably, it taught me a great lesson.

I realized that I didn't really know what I wanted. Strangely enough, it has taken me a long time to become aware of this and decide for myself what I like and don't like. I was comparing myself to others and seeing what they had, wanting this for myself. Then when I would get it, I was miserable, realizing I didn't really want it in the first place. I changed my mind constantly. I could never tell my wife what I wanted for my birthday or Father's Day, since I really didn't know what I wanted.

I found out that my motives in almost everything I did were totally selfish and self-centered. I wanted to be accepted by everybody I knew and to be the most popular person at the same time. The face I would put on would depend on where I was, and with whom I hung out.

If you hated somebody, I gossiped about that person too. If you loved somebody, then they were my best friend too. I could never make decisions for myself either. It's no wonder I was so miserable. It takes a lot of effort to please everybody and fit into every situation.

I had been stuffing my emotions with food for years. I was waiting for somebody to give me that opportunity, that chance at life. Just sitting waiting for somebody to change me.

In truth, I didn't need anybody to help me. I am the solution just as I am the problem, but I had to stop eating in order to get in touch with my inner self to discover this. Once I started to feel my feelings, I started to become comfortable with myself. With time, I actually liked myself and then really appreciated myself for who I am. I became aware of my defects, as well as my positive traits and talents. I started to have a realistic picture of who I am. I realized that I could make a mistake but that it doesn't mean that I am a mistake.

I also found out that others can and do make mistakes; and I'm cool with that, too. Once I started to like others and me too, then I saw that I could accept everybody just as they are, imperfect human beings.

What transpired was truly amazing; I started to actually love myself. Not in a conceited way, but in a very healthy way. Once that happened, I was not only capable of giving love, but more important, I was capable of receiving love; truly a gift. All those resentments and judgmental attitudes disappeared. I appreciated life for life, and what an awesome life it is.

Today, when self-doubt comes in, I focus on where I used to be, and recognize and acknowledge my accomplishments so far, even if they were minimal in size. They say: "money is the root of all evil." I believe self-doubt is the real root of all evil. When I am in doubt, I am paralyzed. I'm lost and can't move forward. When I am confident, I can conquer worlds.

A friend sent me a quote from Jane Addams a couple of years ago and I keep it posted on my office wall above my computer. It has helped me immensely during those doubtful times. Jane Addams (September 6, 1860 – May 21, 1935) was the daughter of Illinois Senator John Addams. She was truly a remarkable woman who understood that self-doubt is debilitating and that belief in self is the only way to live. Her accomplishments in life included being the first woman to win the Nobel Peace Prize.

I give you her quote with great honor and humility: "Nothing could be worse than the fear that one had given up too soon, and left one unexpended effort that might have saved the world".

Take a moment and let these words sink into your heart. If I had given up, I would be dead today from obesity or diabetes. I would have never gone to nursing school. I would have never studied about diabetes, and surely would never have studied about cortisol, and the ramifications of its release in the body. It has helped me so much in my personal diabetic care.

A friend of mine who had sought my advice for his own weight loss died while I was writing this book from a heart attack at age forty-two. He left behind a wife with six children: both his parents are still alive. His oldest child is eighteen; the youngest is only three years old.

I tried to help him, but he refused to believe that it was possible for him to lose weight. He would say: "Alan, it's true what you say about my attitude toward food and life, but I'm just too busy. It sounds good and you look great, but I'll never be able to do it." His excuses, his refusal to believe, his denial of the facts, unfortunately cost him his life. He gave up hope and the result was not just tragic, it was fatal. This could have been my story if I had given up hope too.

His sad story and the strong lesson is no joke. You, dear readers, are people who don't need to die. The solution to life is available to us all. Don't give up hope; it takes time, it takes effort, it takes the willingness to stick with the solution that works. Don't despair; it will work for you too.

It's your choice: to live in happiness and joy, free of the dreaded consequences of untreated diabetes, or to die a diabetic death. The choice to live is here for you today. Yes, right now you can choose to be Awesome.

"I call heaven and earth to witness this day against you, that I have set before thee life and death, blessing and cursing; therefore choose life, that both thou and thy seed may live" (Deut. 30:19 jbt)

I promised you in the first chapter that your life would be wonderful if you followed the suggestions in this book. I live an awesome life today simply by focusing on life with a positive attitude. This is the choice I make each time I choose between positive living versus diabetic hell.

I believe that an awesome life is attainable for you, too, in every aspect of your life. Whatever you feel is lacking in your life today, be it health matters, financial difficulties, or relationship struggles, the solution is available for you. Take charge of your life, believe in yourself, and take the necessary actions to live better. You only get one life to live. Make it the best life possible.

REFERENCES

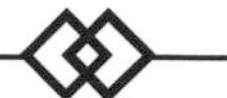

Ausems MG, Verbiest J, Hermans MP, et al (September 1999). "Frequency of glycogen storage disease type II in The Netherlands: implications for diagnosis and genetic counselling". Eur. J. Hum. Genet. 7

Berkman, James; Rifkin, Harold (1973). "Unilateral nodular diabetic glomerulosclerosis (Kimmelstiel-Wilson): Report of a case" Metabolism (Elsevier Inc.)

Brunner & Suddarth 2007 Textbook of Medical-Surgical Nurs- ing Smeltzer, Bare, Hinkle, Cheever 11th Edition Lipincott Williams & Wilkins

Chambers, J.W.; Georg, R.H. and Bass, A.D. (1965) "Effect of Hydrocortisone and Insulin on Uptake of Alpha Aminoisobutyric Acid by Isolated Perfused Rat Liver".

Cryer PE: Hypoglycemia, Pathophysiology, Diagnosis and Treatment, New York, Oxford Univ Press, 1997.

DavidKatzMD.com

DJ Jenkins et al (1981). "Glycemic index of foods: a physiological basis for carbohydrate exchange."

Gorbman, A.; Dickhoff, W.W.; Vigna, S.R.; Clark, N.B.; Muller, A.F,. "Comparative Endocrinology". John Wiley and Sons, New York

Görges, R.; Knappe, G.; Gerl, H.; Ventz, M.; Stahl, F. (1999). "Di- agnosis of Cushing's syndrome: Re-evaluation of midnight plasma cor- tisol vs urinary free cortisol and low-dose dexamethasone suppression test in a large patient group" Journal of Endocrinological Investigation

Greenwood FC, Landon J, Stamp TCB (1965). "The plasma sugar, free fatty acid, cortisol and growth hormone response to insulin" J Clin Invest

Hellman B, Gylfe E, Grapengiesser E, Dansk H, Salehi A (2007). "[Insulin oscillations--clinically important rhythm. Anti-diabetics should increase the pulsative component of the insulin release]" (in Swedish). Jennifer Ibrahim. e-Medicine, Glycogen-Storage Disease Type II Kertes PJ, Johnson TM, ed (2007) Evidence Based Eye Care Philadelphia, PA: Lippincott Williams & Wilkins

Kikuchi T, Yang HW, Pennybacker M, Ichihara N, Mizutani M, Van Hove JL and Chen YT (1998) Clinical and metabolic correction of Pompe disease by enzyme therapy in acid maltase-deficient quail.

King, Michael W. (2005). Lange Q&A USMLE Step 1 (Sixth ed.).New York: McGraw-Hill, Medical Pub. Division. p. 82

Lewis Heitkemper & Dirksen 2004 Medical-Surgical Nursing Ob-rien, Giddens And Bucher 6th edition Mosby

Ludwig DS. The glycemic index: physiological mechanisms relating to obesity, diabetes, and cardiovascular disease. JAMA[3]. 2002;

MacHemer, R (1995). "The development of pars plana vitrectomy: a personal account". Graefe's Archive for Clinical and Experimental Ophthalmology

Manchester, K.L., Sites of Hormonal Regulation of Protein Metabolism. p. 229, Mammalian Protein [Munro, H.N., Ed.]. Academic Press, New York. p. 273

Melloul D, Marshak S, Cerasi E (2002). Regulation of Insulin Gene Transcription Diabetologia

Nieman LK, Ilias I. Evaluation and treatment of Cushing's syndrome. The Journal of American Medicine. 2005

Mosby's 2006 Dictionary of Medicine, Nursing & Health Professionals Editor: Tamara Myers 7th edition Mosby

Nuval.com

Oz 1999 Healing From The Heart Oz & Ornish 1st Edition Plume

Oz 2008 You, The Owner's Manual Roizen & Oz Updated Exp Edi- tion Morrow

Pike, R.L., and Brown, M. Nutrition: An Integrated Approach, 2nd Edition New York: Wiley. 1975

Prentice Hall 2007 Drug Guide Wilson, Shannon, Shields and Stang. Pearson

PubMed Health Diabetic Neuropathy

Scheinfeld N. Dissecting Cellulitis: A Review 2003;9(1):8

Segal, Arthur C. A Linear Diet Model The College Mathematics Journal, January 1987.

Soffer, L.J.; Dorfman, R.I.; Gabrilove, J.L,. "The Human Adrenal Gland" Febiger, Phil

The National Endocrine and Metabolic Diseases Information Service. July 2008.

VanHelder, W., Radomski, Goode, R. and Casey, K. Hormonal and metabolic response to three types of exercise of equal duration and external work output. Eur. J. of Appl. Physiol. 54:337-342. 1985

Wong MC, Chung JW, Wong TK 2007 Effects of Treatments for Symptoms of Diabetic Neuropathy Systemic Review

Printed in the United States
By Bookmasters